A TIME
TO HEAL

How to Reap the Benefits of Holistic Health

A TIME TO HEAL

DANIEL REDWOOD, D.C.

Foreword by James S. Gordon, M.D.

A.R.E. Press • Virginia Beach • Virginia

A.R.E. Press
Sixty-Eighth & Atlantic Avenue
P.O. Box 656
Virginia Beach, VA 23451-0656   7/95

Library of Congress Cataloging-in-Publication Data
Redwood, Daniel, 1948-
    A time to heal : how to reap the benefits of holistic health / by Daniel Redwood.
        p. cm.
    Includes bibliographical references and index.
    ISBN 87604-310-4
    1. Holistic medicine.   2. Chiropractic.   3. Cayce, Edgar, 1877-1945.   I. Title.
R733.R425 1993
615.5'34—dc20   93-28012

Grateful acknowledgment is made for permission to reprint excerpts from the following:

From *Meaning and Medicine* by Larry Dossey, M.D. Copyright © 1991 by Larry Dossey, M.D. Used by permission of Bantam Books, a division of Bantam Doubleday Dell Publishing Group, Inc.

From *Unconditional Life* by Deepak Chopra. Copyright © 1991 by Deepak Chopra, M.D. Used by permission of Bantam Books, a division of Bantam Doubleday Dell Publishing Group, Inc.

From *Getting Well Again* by O. Carl Simonton, S. Matthews-Simonton, and James Creighton. Copyright © 1978 by O. Carl Simonton and Stephanie Matthews-Simonton. Used by permission of Bantam Books, a division of Bantam Doubleday Dell Publishing Group, Inc.

From *Healing Visualizations* by Gerald Epstein. Copyright © 1989 by Gerald Epstein, M.D. Used by permission of Bantam Books, a division of Bantam Doubleday Dell Publishing Group, Inc.

From *The Edgar Cayce Handbook for Health Through Drugless Therapy* by Harold Reilly and Ruth Brod. Copyright © 1975 by Harold Reilly and Ruth Brod. Reprinted by permission of A.R.E. Press.

From *Between the Lines* by B. Lewis Barnett, Jr., M.D. Copyright © 1989 by B. Lewis Barnett, Jr., M.D. Reprinted by permission of The Society of Teachers of Family Medicine.

From *Natural Health, Natural Medicine* by Andrew Weil, M.D. Copyright © 1990 by Andrew Weil, M.D. Reprinted by permission of Houghton Mifflin Co. All rights reserved.

From *The Edgar Cayce Readings.* Copyright © 1971 by the Edgar Cayce Foundation. Reprinted by permission.

From *The Future of the Body* by Michael Murphy. Copyright © 1992 by Michael Murphy. Reprinted by permission of the author.

From *The Relaxation Response* by Herbert Benson, M.D. Copyright © 1975 by Herbert Benson, M.D. Reprinted by permission of William Morrow and Company, Inc. Reprinted by permission.

Cover design by Beth Miller Redwood/Redwood Tree Ink
Cover illustration by Constance Fahey

For Beth, Reuben, and Jessica
and
Norman and Jewel

To every thing there is a season, and a time to every purpose under heaven:

A time to be born, and a time to die; a time to plant, and a time to reap;

A time to kill, and *a time to heal;* a time to break down, and a time to build up;

A time to weep, and a time to laugh; a time to mourn, and a time to dance;

A time to cast away stones, and a time to gather stones together; a time to embrace, and a time to hold back;

A time to gain, and a time to lose; a time to keep, and a time to let go;

A time to rend, and a time to sew; a time for silence, and a time to speak out;

A time of love, and a time of hate; a time of war, and a time of peace.

Ecclesiastes

Contents

Illustrations

ACKNOWLEDGMENTS

I had the help of many fine people in creating this book:

My wife Beth Miller Redwood, who encouraged me to write the book in the first place, provided well-grounded editorial advice when it was most needed, and designed the beautiful cover and shared every part of this book with me. Beth has been a true blessing in my life. Her spirit of love and generosity has been a source of great inspiration for me.

Charles Masarsky, D.C., a chiropractic researcher, educator, writer, and practitioner, who saved me a great deal of library time by graciously sending a hefty pile of exactly the chiropractic research documentation I needed. He also provided some excellent ideas which helped catalyze my thought process during preparation of the "Foundations of the Chiropractic Model" chapter.

Carl Nelson, D.C., a former schoolmate to whom I owe thanks for pointing me in the direction of Dr. Irwin Korr's research, which helped me immeasurably in writing the chapter about Edgar Cayce's theories on spinal manipulation and manual medicine.

Sandra McLanahan, M.D., a gifted and thoughtful holistic physician, who reviewed the chapters on diet and exercise, and offered both encouragement and helpful information.

Meredith Puryear, an exemplar of the prayerful life, whose advice was of great assistance to me while I was writing the meditation and visualization chapters.

Constance Fahey, a skilled and sensitive artist, whose beautiful painting of a redwood forest adorns the cover. She was able to include all the colors of the rainbow and all the elements of Chinese and Indian medicine—earth, water, fire, air, ether, metal, and wood—to create a truly healing work of art.

Joe Dunn, the editor-in-chief at A.R.E. Press, who displayed a welcome willingness to let me follow my own writer's instincts. I appreciate the freedom this gave me.

Others whose help merits thanks are Francis Sporer, David McMillin, Ned McIntosh, Richard Boyle, Alma Crovatt, Cathy Merchand, John Comerford of Digital Design, and Charles Thomas Cayce.

Thanks also to Lou DeSabla, Mary Kay Reynolds, Bonnie and Robin Raindrop, Bob Smith, Neal Vahle, Ravi Dykema, John Crutcher, Susan Bayliss, Paul Willies, Timothy McClellan, and all the other journal and magazine publishers and editors who have published my writing through the years.

Last, but by no means least, I want to thank three men I met when I was a young adult, who influenced me greatly with their integrity and courage: Clinton Deveaux, David Harris, and César Chavez.

FOREWORD

by James S. Gordon, M.D.

Our health care system is changing. U.S. President Bill Clinton is determined to make health care available to everyone and to cut its cost. Congress agrees. And the American people demand it. But the changes we are seeking involve not just cutting costs and extending coverage. We need a different kind of health care offered in a different spirit.

Doctors are uneasy about the care they give and patients are dissatisfied with the care they receive. Both deplore the brevity of their contact, the lack of feeling and connection, and the paucity of answers for the illnesses that tax all of us. We are wonderful at treating life-threatening emergencies, but we are far less effective in helping the tens of millions of us—doctors and patients alike—who do or will suffer from chronic stress-related illness. Our medicines may relieve or suppress immediate symptoms, but by neglecting the causative factors, they all too often produce serious long-term side effects. We now need not only a new system, but a new way of caring for ourselves and those who come to us for help.

Daniel Redwood—a chiropractor and a healer—is finding his way on this way. He is a confident traveler and a gentle guide. As he takes us with him on his journey toward the new health care, he helps us along on our own.

In *A Time to Heal*, we feel the stirrings of Daniel's desire to help and to heal. We watch as he chooses the hands-on healing of chiropractic to be the vehicle for his wish to be of service. Explaining his choice, he reminds us that manipulation has been a part of all ancient healing traditions, that chiropractic and osteopathy are simply its modern expressions. He succinctly and carefully presents the scientific literature which demonstrates the effectiveness of these therapies in treating back pain, headaches, and menstrual problems, among other medical conditions. And he guides us through the other approaches— including diet, exercise, relaxation, and attitudinal change—which help make chiropractic a vital profession, as well as a helpful technique. Most of all, he shows us how, in the hands of a loving, thoughtful physician, this approach works with the suffering people who come for help.

I finished *A Time to Heal* feeling deeply appreciative. We are in a time when alternative medicines including chiropractic are receiving a long-overdue public and scientific hearing. NIH's newly created Office of Alternative Medicine (on whose Advisory Committee I serve) is exploring the utility of manipulative therapies, as well as acupuncture, nutrition, homeopathy, and other approaches. We are in need of case histories which illustrate the power of these techniques and discussions of research which scientifically demonstrates their effectiveness. We are equally in need of the larger perspective on health and healing which sustains these techniques. And, perhaps most of all, we need models of healers—people who in their practice and in their being are willing to enlarge the prevailing orthodoxy as they serve others.

In his work and the way he writes about it, Dr. Redwood is such a model. This book of his perspective as a chiropractor, *A Time to Heal*, comes at the right time for all of us.

James S. Gordon, M.D.
Washington, D.C.

James Gordon, M.D., is clinical professor in the Departments of Psychiatry and Community and Family Medicine at the Georgetown University School of Medicine, and is the founder and director of the Center for Mind-Body Studies. He is the author of nine books, including the award-winning Health for the Whole Person.

INTRODUCTION

This book is about holistic healing from a chiropractor's perspective.

The holistic paradigm now emergent in our culture recognizes that body, mind, and spirit are indivisible. In my work with more than 3,500 patients from all walks of life over the past fifteen years, I have seen this firsthand.

I have drawn a series of case studies from my practice, with the purpose of illustrating both the healing power of chiropractic and the importance of seeing each patient as a whole person, not as a set of dysfunctional body parts. These stories are not typical; most chiropractic cases are less complex. But each of the stories you are about to read unlocked a door for me, helping me to better understand the healing process. I believe they can also unlock doors for you.

The first story in the book is my own. I have focused on the events that kindled my interest in the healing arts and led me to become a chiropractor. Throughout *A Time to Heal*, I have done my best to demystify chiropractic, explaining it in terms under-standable to the average reader. Chiropractic is both a science and an art; I have tried to present the science without getting too dry and the art without becoming too esoteric.

Encouraging patient empowerment through self-healing methods is an important part of my work. The "Tools for Self-Healing" section offers both scientific information and down-to-earth, practical suggestions for healthier living through diet and nutrition, exercise and yoga, and relaxation and medita-tion. I hope you not only read these chapters, but put them to practical use. That's what they're for.

Particularly in the last half of the book, I have focused on the health information in the Edgar Cayce readings. In my view, Cayce's work represents the most advanced Western holistic syn-thesis of its time (the first half of the twentieth century), and perhaps ours as well. I have presented the Cayce information alongside other systems I respect, noting the areas of agreement as well as those of divergence.

Chiropractic is moving toward integration into the health mainstream in our lifetime. There has long been a rift between chiropractic and mainstream medicine, in which the former has been attacked for lacking scientific research and for being founded on a philosophy which includes ideas such as the exist-ence of an "innate intelligence" as the source of healing.

As this book makes clear, chiropractic now has a solid and growing base of scientific research. In addition, conventional medicine has in recent years come to increasingly recognize the crucial role of mind-body interactions in restoring and maintain-ing health.

I see great value in learning the language of science, respect-ing its worthy contributions, and adding to them. At the same time, I believe it would be a tragic mistake for us to feel that this requires abandoning the fundamentally spiritual viewpoint that inspired our founders. Science and spirituality are not enemies, as Albert Einstein, Thomas Edison, chiropractic's founder Daniel David Palmer, Edgar Cayce, and countless others affirmed in their day.

May we have the vision and the courage to affirm it in ours.

Daniel Redwood, D.C.
Virginia Beach, Virginia
October, 1993

CHAPTER 1

A LONG AND WINDING ROAD: MY STORY

*"Your work is to discover your work
And then with all your heart
To give yourself to it."*
                    Buddha

I didn't grow up intending to be a doctor—until I was well into my twenties, the thought never crossed my mind. For a long time, until several years past my graduation from college, I did my best to avoid committing to any traditional career track. I came of age in the sixties, and I took very seriously that part of the American dream which says that freedom is the road on which life is most fully lived. Deep in my heart, that's still how I feel.

I think that all of us in the natural healing arts have a touch of the rebel in us. We may be unremarkable or even conformist in many aspects of our lives, but those who lack all willingness to sail against the wind choose other professions. To be in this field, you've got to be willing to stand up for what you believe in, even in the face of determined opposition.

Songwriter-poet Ric Masten, when he gave a concert for the student body at my chiropractic college, said we were the first group he'd met that had freely chosen to become members of a minority group. And while the challenges of being a chiropractor can by no stretch of the imagination be considered equivalent to those that come with membership in a racial or ethnic minority, I know what my old friend Ric meant.

The common ground, as I see it, is this: both chiropractors and minorities know what it's like to feel the sting of unjust criticism, and we learn early on that unless we strengthen ourselves in response, we will break under the pressure.

My life has been marked by so many unexpected turns in the road that I've developed something of a distrust for long-term planning. It has sometimes seemed to me that whoever's writing my life's script has a deeply ironic sense of humor, coupled with an unexcelled knack for teaching difficult lessons well.

I was born in a hospital in New York City in 1948, and it was three days before my mother was allowed to hold me. I suspect that this contributed to my becoming ill almost immediately. From my earliest days, I struggled with eczema, allergies, and asthma.

Since I was the first-born child and my father was an excellent photographer, there are many photos in our family albums showing me as an infant. Once, as an adult, I was nostalgically thumbing through the pages of one of these albums and was struck by the fact that in some pictures my eyes are bright with wonder, while in others I look extremely dazed. When I asked my mother about this, she replied without a moment's hesitation, "Oh, that must have been when you were taking your medication."

I knew that I had taken medication a great deal, but not until I saw the contrast between the drugged and undrugged photographs did I grasp what a drain the whole process had been. If you're a child and that's all you know, I guess it seems normal.

"People used to say you looked like you had a light bulb inside your head," my mother recalled, "but you didn't look the same when you took your medicine." This is an understatement. I looked like a zombie. Whatever light bulb may have been there was definitely switched off by the medication.

My parents grew up in the era when the "wonder drugs" were developed. Seeing contagious diseases, which had killed thousands upon thousands of people a generation earlier, miraculously controlled by antibiotics, they were grateful beyond words. When I developed physical ailments, they sought help from mainstream medical physicians. Mixed in with many happy memories from my childhood are recollections of dozens upon dozens of visits to doctors, countless spoonfuls and tablets of medicine, and an ongoing vague sense that something could go wrong at any time.

Asthma was particularly frightening because it threatened my very ability to breathe. I recall many a night when I was unable to take a full deep breath. We would build a "tent" of blankets on my bed, and as the moist mist from a vaporizer filled the tent, I would sit inside it, propped up on a few pillows, wheezing until I fell asleep. This must have been a very trying experience for my parents, but to their credit they never blamed me. They just tried to do everything they could to help.

For the most part, I had what I consider a good, normal childhood and didn't feel disabled by my illnesses. I played baseball, basketball, and football with varying degrees of success, did well at school, and on the whole didn't get into much trouble.

When I was ten, trouble got into me. On a chilly February night, as my father and I were getting ready to go to Madison Square Garden to watch the track and field championships, I got sicker than I had ever been before or have been since. My breathing became labored and painful very quickly, with each breath a greater challenge than the one before. When my father told me we were skipping the track meet, I knew I had something serious.

It was a combination of pneumonia and pleurisy, an infection of the lungs and the fluid-filled sacs that surround them. Our family doctor made a Saturday night housecall, God bless him, and gave me a shot of penicillin with a long needle in my rear end, after which he stayed for an hour or two to be certain I was responding.

My parents told me later that if I had had the same problem forty years earlier, I would almost certainly have died, like thousands of others in the great epidemics. As I recall, they waited until I had fully recovered before sharing this bit of history with me, so as not to tempt fate.

From this episode, I learned a healthy respect for Western medicine. When it comes to saving lives threatened by acute infectious illnesses, I have not seen anything that surpasses it.

Though I later spent years taking advanced science courses, by junior high I was almost completely turned off by science classes. I memorized the material and got A's on most of the tests, but by the eighth grade my native curiosity had been pretty thoroughly washed away. I remember a conversation with my parents, in which I told them how we were learning about electricity at school. I had all the definitions down pat, everything about AC and DC and ohms and watts, but I still couldn't understand what electricity *was*.

"But what exactly *is* it?" I recall asking them. "What makes it move?" Unfortunately, neither my parents nor my science teacher were able to answer that question to my satisfaction. From that day until the time I decided to go to chiropractic school at age twenty-eight, I never put my heart into another science course. I took them and did well, but it was all rote learning and of little interest to me. As soon as I was allowed to stop taking science courses, I did so.

What was it that turned me off? I think the question is worth pursuing, because I am certain the same thing happens to most American students before they reach high school. The problem I had perceived, in my own naïve way, was that science (at least the way it is taught in most schools) does not go to the heart of existence. It cannot fully explain the world in which we live. Beyond what science can explain, there is a vaster realm of mystery.

If someone had just told me that back in junior high, that person would have done me a great favor. It would have given me confidence that my questions were worthwhile and valid and had also been pondered by great scientists. Furthermore, I believe it would have encouraged in me a more understanding and, therefore, patient frame of mind, with which I could more fruitfully have approached my science classes. In truth, it is no criticism of science to acknowledge that while it is an excellent tool for explaining many things, large parts of life fall outside its purview.

But no one told me that, so I said good-by to science and gravitated to the liberal arts. In college at the State University of New York at Buffalo, I majored in English, focusing on contemporary writers, poets, and political theorists. I was elected to a leadership position in the university's student government and was one of the school's delegates to the National Student Association Congress. I had one close friend who was a biology major (he later became a holistic dentist), but just about everyone else I knew was in the humanities or the social sciences.

I also played the guitar for hours a day, sang in a jug band called The South Happiness Street Society Skiffle Band that toured northern New York State and southern Canada, and in general did my best to immerse myself in the swirling cultural currents of that now-mythical time called the sixties.

In early 1971, I moved to the San Francisco area and worked for several months at a health food store, which awakened my interest in learning about natural healing methods. At the same time, I pursued my singing and songwriting career. It wasn't much of a career by Hollywood standards, but I did a great deal of singing for causes I believed in (including a tour around the country in support of the United Farmworkers Union lettuce boycott), and gave my all to seeing how far the music would take me.

In 1972, I was a traveling musician on the road. I performed at schools, churches, synagogues, union halls, conferences, folk festivals, and on radio and television. This brought me very little money, but a great deal of satisfaction, the kind that comes from doing something you believe in. I had long dreamed of making music on a full-time basis. As things turned out, that was the only time in my life I actually did it.

The main lesson I learned was that it is very important to follow your dreams, whatever the result. As long as you do, you won't be looking back over your shoulder twenty or thirty years later, wondering "What if?"

One night in Buffalo, passing through my former hometown on a singing tour that went from California to New York and back again, I stayed over at the home of a friend's mother. I have always been an avid reader, and when I saw some well-stocked bookshelves in the den, I scanned the titles in search of something exciting and unfamiliar. I spotted a book called *The Sleeping Prophet*, found its title and cover intriguing, and dove right in. I couldn't put it down for hours.

The book, which had been a best seller for author Jess Stearn several years earlier, is a biography of Edgar Cayce, who had the uncanny ability to enter an altered state and access information far beyond his waking knowledge. Until his death in 1945, he used this talent primarily to diagnose and suggest treatments for the thousands of ailing people who sought his help.

Cayce's story touched me deeply. I have always been moved by stories of people who seem more interested in serving others than in accumulating personal power and wealth, and Edgar Cayce was clearly one of these. I also have an ongoing fascination with probing the outer limits of human potential, and Cayce's abilities more than piqued my curiosity in this regard. Furthermore, natural healing methods were by then among my main interests, and the Cayce readings on this subject presented information at a higher level of integration than I had found elsewhere.

Over the next year, I read dozens of books on both Cayce and natural healing, pursuing what has become a continuing quest for greater understanding. I sought out books on herbs, foods, vitamins and minerals, bodywork of all sorts, and on the connection among body, mind, and spirit. *The Sleeping Prophet* catalyzed my growth process, pointing me in new directions that changed the course of my life.

Not long after returning to the West Coast, I moved to Los Angeles, convinced that if I were ever to have my big break in the recording industry, I had to be near Hollywood. I got a "day job" at a health food store near the beach in Venice and continued to play music in my off hours.

At first, most of my time at the store was spent stocking shelves and ringing up items on the register. This was a learning experience in more ways than one. An honors student and university graduate, I now got a firsthand view of what it was like to work at a low-paying, nonprofessional job. It was particularly instructive to see how some people treated me as an equal, while others (I am glad to say there were fewer of them) looked down on me as their presumed inferior. I have never forgotten what that felt like.

Working in the health food store, I met many people for whom natural healing methods were a way of life. There was an elderly Russian immigrant whose arthritis was controlled by daily doses of a mixture of royal jelly and honey, "just like in the old country," and several people for whom regular intake of cherry juice appeared to have the same effect. There was one young man who came in a couple of times a week to buy a half-gallon of fresh carrot juice and organic vegetables. His doctors had told him several years earlier that he would be dead from cancer within six months, so he decided to become his own doctor.

The store also attracted Hollywood stars like Burgess Meredith and Jane Fonda, who would stop by to stock up on healthful foods, and the weight lifters from Gold's Gym, just down the block, who would drop in after their workouts to recharge with fresh juices and organic fruits. One of the weight lifters, the tall one with the unmistakable muscles and the big smile, was then-unknown Arnold Schwarzenegger.

The owner of the store was a student at Los Angeles College of Chiropractic, and sometimes when the store wasn't too busy, he talked with me at length about two of his great passions—nutrition and chiropractic. Working at that store also provided me with the reason for my first-ever visit to a chiropractor, after I injured my lower back lifting a crate of juice the wrong way. Fortunately, workers' compensation covered chiropractic care, and the treatment I received helped me toward a swift recovery.

While living in Los Angeles, I had frequent bouts of bronchitis. The infamous L.A. smog, superimposed on my already delicate upper respiratory tract, made for chronic difficulty. One day, a friend said he was going camping in the Sierra Nevada Mountains and promised to bring me some mountain-grown yerba santa herb when he returned. He was true to his word, and I made a tea from the fragrant leaves of the plant. After drinking it for a few days, my bronchitis, which had been bothering me for several weeks straight, vanished without a trace. I was impressed.

I remained symptom-free until several months later, when the problem returned. Since I didn't know anyone who was going to the Sierras at that point, I figured I could cure myself with the packaged yerba santa we sold at the store. But when I opened the package, the leaves were older and dryer and had no fragrance. They also had no therapeutic effect whatsoever.

From this I learned that one batch of an herb is not necessarily the same as another batch. Since plants are not manufactured in laboratories, they vary greatly in effectiveness. Freshness is an all-important quality, as I later read in French herbalist Maurice Messegué's book, *Of People and Plants*. Since then I have learned that herbal potency can be retained by methods such as freeze-drying or alcohol extraction, but it does fade quickly if the leaves or roots are cut up and left exposed to the air.

One day in the health food store, I started thinking about going to chiropractic school. It offered me the chance to use what I was learning about natural healing, to do something of value for others, to make a good living, and to be my own boss. But I understood that this would mean a full-time, long-term commitment, and I still wasn't ready to abandon my dream of a singing career.

Two years later, after a Hollywood recording contract on which I had placed high hopes fell through and after teaching English and math to ninth and tenth graders turned out to be a less than idyllic experience, I was ready. In early 1977, after taking the prerequisite college science courses, I enrolled at Palmer College of Chiropractic in Davenport, Iowa.

Palmer provided me with a solid chiropractic education, as well as a sense of living tradition. Founded around the turn of the century by Daniel David Palmer, the discoverer of chiropractic, the institution had grown and matured over several decades.

By the time I arrived in the 1970s, the basic science courses were taught by master's and doctorate degree holders from universities, and the quality of all coursework and clinical training was monitored by the Council on Chiropractic Education, an accrediting agency which, in turn, was accredited by the federal government. Chiropractic had come a long way from its humble beginnings. Chiropractors were licensed in all fifty states and many foreign countries, and the movement toward the mainstream was well under way.

Yet with all the changes, Palmer remained deeply steeped in tradition. Unlike some other chiropractic institutions, Palmer College was extremely reluctant to allow any perceived dilution of traditional chiropractic. This meant that the use of physical therapy machines, such as ultrasound or electronic muscle stimulators, and the use of vitamin, mineral, and herbal supplements were strongly discouraged. The school considered these outside the chiropractor's legitimate scope of practice, even though most state laws allowed chiropractors to employ these methods.

The school's policy ran directly counter to my own inclinations, and I later opposed it in one especially uncomfortable meeting with school administrators when I was student body president. Yet, in retrospect, I feel that I benefited from the strictures it imposed. Because we were discouraged from using physical therapy machines and nutritional supplements, we learned firsthand the powerful healing effects of hands-on chiropractic adjustments. When the adjustment is the only therapy employed and the healing response is dramatic, there can be little doubt as to the cause-and-effect relationship, particularly when good responses occur in case after case.

At Palmer, I saw both strengths and weaknesses in conservative adherence to chiropractic tradition. One major strength was that we students were constantly exposed to faculty members and field doctors who had seen the healing power of pure chiropractic time and again and had internalized these experiences as the bedrock core of their healing philosophy. "Find it, fix it, and leave it alone," we were told, referring to the spinal subluxation (a joint dysfunction with nerve irritation) and corrective manual adjustment that together constitute the centerpiece of chiropractic's contribution to the healing arts.

There is a focused simplicity to that statement which I find quite appealing. The "leave it alone" part, in particular, shows a respect for the healing power of the body and, ultimately, the limitations of outside intervention. Not only chiropractors but all health practitioners would be well advised to heed this more often.

We were also taught at Palmer that there is an "innate intelligence" within us that is the source of all healing and that "the power that made the body heals the body." These spiritual conceptions of physical healing have brought condemnation upon chiropractors at times, but now, in the late twentieth century, it is widely understood that healing does not occur solely on a physical level.

Chiropractic philosophy, as taught at Palmer, also emphasized basic principles in the common domain shared by all natural healing arts. Profound and deceptively simple, these ideas are ignored far more frequently than they are practiced.

They include:

- eating natural foods
- eating only when you are hungry
- drinking only when you are thirsty
- sleeping when you are tired

Simple, yes? Yet I have almost never met anyone who follows all of these recommendations, and, as far as I can see, most people don't follow any of them consistently. But rather than kick ourselves too hard for our imperfections, a good place to begin the change is by acknowledging that these are worthy ideals and making a commitment to do the right thing more of the time.

In our busy modern lives, who among us really eats according to hunger rather than according to the clock? How many of us stop eating when we are full and drink only when we are thirsty? And how often do we push ourselves when tired, in order to catch up with all the responsibilities that continually weigh upon us? I, for one, would have to plead guilty on a number of counts.

Natural healing philosophy and the branch of that tree known as chiropractic philosophy call for a more sane and balanced way of life. This is not easily lived up to, but it is well worth the effort. We need to take small and, when possible, large steps to reorient our approach to health. All worthwhile philosophies call us to stretch beyond our current conceptions of our possibilities. Chiropractic, with the more natural way of life its ideals embody, is no exception.

One weakness of traditional chiropractic, I observed early on, was a tendency among some of its adherents to a close-mindedness when it came to seeing the value in healing methods other than their own. This is not a failing unique to chiropractors, but I found it disturbing nonetheless.

Seeing this helped strengthen my own resolve to learn what I could about a wide range of other approaches to healing. I wanted to understand their strengths and weaknesses, so that I could utilize those which meshed well with my chiropractic methods and refer patients to other practitioners when that was likely to be helpful. Aside from the patients I have referred to medical specialists such as radiologists, neurosurgeons, and orthopedic surgeons, my most frequent referrals over the years have been to massage therapists and acupuncturists. Both of these healing arts are still very much underutilized by the population at large, as is chiropractic, but this is changing for the better.

I have long had an attraction to the cultures and healing arts of Asia. While I have read extensively about acupuncture and have been treated with it as well, my personal portal of entry into the Eastern healing arts came through a course in polarity therapy which I attended at Palmer.

Dr. Ed Jarvis, who taught the course, had a profound effect on me. I felt a strong generational and cultural connection with this young California chiropractor, who was the finest healer I had seen. In addition, I was very attracted to the course material, which was based on the work of Dr. Randolph Stone, a chiropractor and osteopath who had brought it back from India.

Polarity therapy assumes that body, mind, and spirit are an indivisible whole. Thus physical symptoms are perceived to have meaning in terms of the patient's overall life patterns. This viewpoint is common to all of the Eastern healing arts, but it is anathema to much of modern Western medicine and even runs counter to some of the dominant trends in contemporary chiropractic.

Therein lies the crux of the tale that follows. Since taking Dr. Jarvis' course, I have never been able to easily view physical symptoms in strictly physical terms. Back pain can come from a spinal subluxation, a strained muscle, or a sprained ligament, yes, but if we cone down our vision too tightly, we miss deeper levels of causation—the feeling of failure at work or in a marriage, the frustration of not having followed one's dreams, or the sense that life has become devoid of meaning.

One of the main claims historically made by many chiropractors is that in finding and correcting spinal subluxations, we are correcting the cause of disease or "dis-ease." I think this is true, but only up to a point. Bringing structural balance to the body and thereby allowing it to function more properly is, in fact, working at a deeper level of causation than methods which suppress symptoms with medication. But from where I stand, it is an act of supreme hubris to claim that correcting spinal subluxations gets to the deepest levels of causation. It is no admission of failure on our part to acknowledge this. The deepest levels of causation are probably beyond the reach of any technique, no matter how brilliant its conception or impressive its lineage.

These levels can be accessed, but the path is never fully predictable and a technique that works one time may fail the next. In my opinion, healers who see their methods as the end point, the omega, of the evolution of the human healing arts would do well to think again. We are nowhere near the omega. We are only granted occasional glimpses.

It is a basic human trait to try to plumb the meaning of our experiences, to dig below the surface to elicit the hidden gold within. Yet it is important, as we mine the inner veins of theory and imagination, not to lose our close connection with the outer world that grounds our quest.

The poet Novalis said, "The seat of the soul is where the inner world and the outer world meet." One thing I particularly appreciate about day-in, day-out work with patients is that it requires constantly translating the philosophical into the practical, the inner into the outer, and thus keeps me from drifting too far into a primarily mental mode of functioning.

The life of another great poet, William Carlos Williams, a physician from Paterson, New Jersey, provides a model of this kind of balance. Williams moved back and forth between seeing patients and creating great poetry, a remarkable blend of skills. Doctoring has a way of adding earth to a poet's fire, air, and water. In my own writing, I, too, make an effort to ground my speculations in the earth of experience.

Since my days at Palmer College, I have never gone too long without also grounding myself in the push-and-pull of professional politics. When I was student body president at Palmer, I arranged for us to invite Congressman James Corman of California to address the students and faculty. Corman was co-author of the Corman-Stone Law, which had legislated chiropractic inclusion in Medicare several years earlier and was the House sponsor of the Kennedy-Corman bill, which at the time was the leading legislative vehicle for proponents of national health insurance.

I asked him to speak on the role of government in health care, and he gave a thought-provoking speech which called on all of us to recognize the need for a system in which no one would be denied the health care he or she needed. The son of a Kansas lead miner who died young, Jim Corman remembered what it was like to be one of the downtrodden and believed simple justice required helping those most in need. We were inspired and, frankly, relieved to see that we as chiropractors had support not only in our own small circles, but among senior members of Congress as well.

I spent many hours with Congressman Corman during his day-and-a-half visit to Davenport, and by the end of the visit he had invited me to come to Washington when I graduated, to set up an office near Capitol Hill. He said he would be my first patient and would send his friends.

This was heady stuff. Up to that point, I had planned to practice in a mellow college town in New England. But the congressman's invitation changed my perspective. I rethought my plans (which took about two hours), and set my sights on Washington, D.C.

But there was a catch. When I checked into the procedure for securing a license in the District of Columbia, I discovered that it was the one jurisdiction on the North American continent where no new chiropractic licenses were being granted. It had been more than fifteen years since the last one was issued. Chiropractic was legal in the District and had been since the 1920s, but there were only two chiropractors left in the whole city, both over the age of sixty. The medical board, which controlled the licensing process, refused to allow chiropractic applicants to be tested. The reason for this was never publicly stated, but the longstanding antipathy toward chiropractic by much of organized medicine certainly played a role.

My mind was set on moving to the D.C. area by this time, so I started looking for associateships in chiropractic offices in northern Virginia. None were available, so I started out on my own and have practiced that way ever since. My first office was in Falls Church, Virginia, several miles outside Washington. I saw patients there on Tuesday nights, Thursday nights, and Saturday mornings at the start, while working full-time during the week as director of special projects for the International Chiropractors Association (ICA), which was headquartered in downtown Washington. Congressman Corman was true to his word and became one of my first patients.

My first office may have set the world's record for "smallest office, chiropractor." It was 315 square feet, which meant I had a waiting room and a treatment/consultation room, and that was it. Not even a closet. It cost me $275 a month (including utilities and janitorial services), was located in a well-kept building in a nice town, and was in keeping with my belief that a practice should grow organically and start as debt-free as possible.

My first year in practice, I wrote an article that was published in the *International Review of Chiropractic*, telling new graduates how to set up an office on a shoestring. Unlike newly minted medical physicians, who can get jobs in hospitals or public clinics, chiropractors at this stage of our profession's evolution really have no options other than starting a practice from scratch or working as an associate in someone else's private practice. Many of the new chiropractic graduates of my era (it may still be true) assumed that the only way to set up an office on their own was to secure a substantial bank loan and then begin with a large, fully staffed, high-tech operation from day one. While that may be the best choice for those who desire that kind of practice and can arrange the financing, I wanted everyone to know there were other possibilities. Not as glamorous perhaps, but offering far more independence than an associateship and much less debt than the bank loan route.

After I had practiced in Falls Church for three years, the District of Columbia changed its rules (under threat of a lawsuit and with some expert lobbying) to allow a reasonable licensing procedure, and the next year I moved my practice to Sixteenth and K Streets, four blocks from the White House. The District is a dynamic place, with fascinating people from all over the world. I enjoyed the variety and intensity of the city and loved driving past the Lincoln Memorial and the Washington Monument on the way to work every day. That never got old.

The rich and the poor, the powerful and the humble, often sat next to each other in my reception room. An aching back is a great equalizer, I discovered. My patients ranged from famous leaders of Congress to the inner-city unemployed. Each of them had something to teach me. I have always felt that getting to know my patients is as rewarding a part of my practice as the physical healing work, and I suspect that part of what helps my patients get well is our conversations, even the parts when we're not talking about their health problems.

There is something about this kind of old-time country-doctor approach that feels like home to me, even in the middle of a city. I don't like to rush, and consequently I enjoy my practice most when the schedule is only moderately full, rather than jammed from morning to night.

During my years in Washington, I started to write on a regular basis. It began with an article on chiropractic for *Pathways*, a holistically oriented community magazine. Soon, I was writing quarterly book and music review columns for them, and within a couple of years I started doing extended interviews with people like Marilyn Ferguson, Larry Dossey, Deepak Chopra, John Bradshaw, Elisabeth Kübler-Ross, Charles Thomas Cayce, Raymond Moody, and many more.

These articles were picked up by alternative papers around the country, and soon I had what seemed like a little cottage industry going. It was a true labor of love, bringing in little income and taking a great deal of time. Looking back on it all, I feel that this writing was, and is, one of the most enjoyable things I've ever done. It has enabled me to meet and converse with some of my personal heroes and has certainly forced me to clarify my own thinking. This book is in a very real sense an outgrowth of the writing I've done for *Pathways*, and I have drawn on the *Pathways* interviews at various points in this book.

More than once in Washington, I had patients tell me I didn't have "urban vibes" or that they were surprised to find someone like me in the heart of the downtown. It took a while for this native New Yorker to admit it, but I eventually concluded that they were right. One day, as I was driving to work in the morning rush hour, I asked myself if I could envision doing the same thing for the next thirty years. I knew immediately that the answer was no and that it was just a question of when I would move. Within a year, I sold my practice and moved to Virginia Beach, a block from the ocean—to the land of seagull, pelican, bald cypress, and live oak.

It's been an eventful journey, and the winds of change keep blowing.

STORIES OF HEALING

CHAPTER 2

TWENTY YEARS OF HEADACHES

I was warned from the start that Jimmy didn't like going to doctors. His cousin, a patient of mine, had been telling me for months about Jimmy's famous headaches, the ones no doctor had been able to cure in twenty years. Like most people who have been to dozens of doctors without lasting relief for pain, Jimmy was tired of even trying. He came to me in desperation.

A hardworking, thirty-six-year-old contractor, he seemed friendly though somewhat jittery when he first walked into my consultation room. He maintained good eye contact as we spoke, and I sensed at least a dim ray of hope present within him. Otherwise, he wouldn't have made the fifteen-mile trip to my office at the end of a long work day. Long days on the job were routine for Jimmy, often involving heavy lifting and having to twist his body into uncomfortable positions for extended periods of time. Physical stress like this is tough for any body to endure for very long, but for Jimmy it was often excruciating.

Back in high school, Jimmy loved football. An excellent running back and a safety, he hit opponents hard and expected the same from them. What he didn't expect was an injury that would plague him throughout his adult life. At age sixteen, a time when many young men believe themselves to be indestructible, Jimmy discovered otherwise. In the middle of one game, while he was running with the ball, he slipped and fell flat on his back. At first, there seemed to be no problem. He shook it off and kept playing. But when he awoke the next morning, his neck hurt like nothing he had ever experienced or even imagined before.

Jimmy recalls it this way:

"During the game, it didn't even hurt at all. Hardly knocked the wind out of me. I thought that I was really going to be hurt bad, but I didn't feel anything. Then I woke up the next morning screaming at the top of my lungs. It felt as if somebody were taking a great big giant vise and crushing the bones in my neck.

"This was my first experience with *bad* pain. So my parents took me to the doctor, and he put a neck brace on. He said, 'You'll be fine. You had some vertebrae moved around, and tossing in your sleep you moved them some more. That's why you're pinching a nerve.' I wore the collar for three months. Then they took it off and said, 'You're fine! You're healed!' As far as I knew, I was. I felt great. I was a sixteen-year-old kid. What the heck did I know?"

Things went well for about a year. Then one day at school, that all changed quickly:

"It was in English class, and each of us had to get up and read a book report in front of the class. As I listened to other people read their reports, I started to feel a sharp pain on one side of my head. As the class went on, by the time it was my turn to get up there and do it, my head was absolutely killing me. I remember my report was on *Huckleberry Finn*. I could hardly make it through. I rushed through it fast as the wind just to get it over with, so I could sit back down.

Then I put my head on the desk and hoped it would go away."

This was no normal, garden-variety headache and was a harbinger of things to come:

"I knew at the time that it didn't feel like a regular headache. I had had headaches before, the ones across the forehead. This didn't feel anything like that. It was hurting me really bad, but then it stopped after about an hour, just like a switch had gone off. I felt fine for maybe a week or so, and then it happened again. From that point on, it started happening about every other day. It was getting more frequent and more intense.

"Finally, my parents said, 'Something's definitely wrong here,' and they took me to an eye-ear-nose-and-throat doctor, because my sinuses would pack up during an attack. He checked me out and told me I had an allergy. He said, 'We're going to put you on this pill. And that will stop the headache.'

"So I started taking these tiny yellow pills, Sansert®. Sure enough, they stopped the headaches, by opening up the blood vessels in my head. But they made me so sick to my stomach that I threw up everything I ate each time I took one. So I said, 'Forget this, I'm not going to take them!' And oddly enough, if I remember correctly, I didn't get the headaches for a while after I stopped taking them."

Why was that?

"It turned out to be because of the warm weather. They had taken me to that doctor in the early spring, when I was seventeen. And then, when the warm weather came, I didn't have the headaches any more, even without the pills. Didn't have a headache all through that summer. Then around October it started getting cold, and the headaches returned. I started taking codeine pills and any other kind of pills I could get my hands on. Anything to stop it. Bottles and bottles of Excedrin®. One time I OD'd on codeine so badly I was kind of like unconscious, but talking, for three days.

"I was so out of it that I didn't even relate any of it to the headache, to the fact that I had taken all those codeine pills because I hurt. I would take anything—antihistamines, analgesics, anything I could find, just to stop the headache. I was loaded, all the time. This continued all through the winter. Then with the very first breaths of warm air in the spring, the headaches stopped."

But Jimmy had started a habit that was hard to break:

"I got married at nineteen, and my wife went to work for a doctor. She could bring home all kinds of stuff. I stayed drugged all through that next winter. By spring, I didn't want to stop. Headache or no headache, the medication felt great, and I wanted to stay on it. These were samples the doctors give, and with my wife working in a doctor's office, I could have all I wanted. Six, seven, eight a day. Never run out. I don't know how my body took that. I was young! I had horrible diet habits, and I lived on those pills."

As the years went by, Jimmy's headaches gradually increased in frequency and intensity, and he continued to take painkillers as a regular part of his day. This was partly out of concern that a sharp, stabbing headache might hit at any moment and partly to help with the neck, shoulder, and upper back pain he had developed, which was less severe than the headaches, though more persistent.

By the time he came to see me at age thirty-six, even though on medication, Jimmy was having regular episodes of what his medical physician diagnosed as cluster headaches, which frequently took him to the hospital emergency room.

"I really resisted going to the hospital. I mean, at first I thought, 'This is too ridiculous!' To call the ambulance for a headache? But my wife, my second wife, said, 'I'm calling them!'

"Those headaches, the ones bad enough to send me to the hospital, they felt as though someone were driving a nail into this spot right in front of my ear. A nail that didn't have any end, that just kept going. Bang! Bang! Over and over. I don't even like to think about this any more."

Headaches can arise from a variety of causes. Many patients, Jimmy among them, exhibit a combination of these causative factors. The nervous system and circulatory system are the keys to understanding headaches.

The nervous system is involved in two ways. First, vertebral subluxations disrupt normal nerve transmission, which can adversely affect all areas of the body served by the involved nerves. Where headaches are involved, the vertebrae of the neck are the most common culprits. Second, emotional stress is readily transmitted via the nervous system to the muscles, causing them to increase in tension. When the tension reaches a high enough level, pain begins. Muscles in the neck, head, face, and jaw all can cause headaches.

Moreover, the circulatory and nervous systems are intimately related to each other. The sympathetic nervous system (SNS), the body's "fight-or-flight" stress-response mechanism, functions as a link between the two. The SNS, which has its origin in the lumbar, dorsal, and lower cervical regions of the spine (from the small of the back to the lower neck), controls the nerve supply to the body's blood vessels. Unless normal signal patterns are transmitted by these nerves, the circulatory system will not behave normally. In many cases where spinal manipulation eliminates headaches, it is because balance has been restored to the sympathetics, thus normalizing blood flow to the head.

In general, headaches which focus in the temporal region (near the "temples") are considered to be "vascular headaches," whose primary cause is circulatory. Headaches centered in the neck and back of the head are called "tension headaches" and considered to be primarily muscular. Most headache sufferers have one or the other, but I have seen patients with both at the same time. In both cases—vascular and tension headaches—the spine and the nervous system play crucial roles.

I have seen hundreds of headache sufferers helped by chiropractic. For some, the relief is instant and permanent, as was the case with one young woman who had had constant tension headaches for five years. For others, the recovery is gradual, and during occasional recurrences at times of high stress further chiropractic treatment is required.

Recent research has demonstrated that spinal manipulation is highly effective in relieving headaches. In the preliminary results of a controlled study where chiropractic adjustments were given to one group of headache sufferers, and amitriptyline, a commonly employed prescription headache medication was given to another group, the two groups achieved equal levels of pain relief. But the chiropractic patients maintained their levels of improvement after treatment was stopped, while those treated with medication returned to their pre-treatment status in an average of four weeks.[1]

When I met Jimmy on the day of our first visit, he was juggling five different medications at the same time, including painkillers, steroids, muscle relaxants, and lithium, a drug which can be prescribed for cluster headaches or bipolar disorder (manic-depressive illness). He had recently gone to the hospital with a severe attack and was worried that another might come at any time. His upper arm hurt constantly and felt weak, and his headaches were starting to scare the daylights out of him. On his patient information form, he wrote that he had extreme pain in the head, neck, and upper back, capitalizing and underlining the word "extreme" to make sure I got the message. As we spoke with each other at the initial consultation, he described his neck pain in graphic terms, saying it felt as if someone were "holding it with a firmly gripped pair of pliers." His headaches were severe enough that he mentioned occasionally contemplating suicide.

When I examined Jimmy, he winced and jerked away involuntarily when I pressed on certain areas of his neck, upper back, and shoulders. Fortunately his reflexes, muscle strength, and response to pinpricks were normal, which along with other test results indicated that there was no severe nerve damage in his neck. He had also recently had a magnetic resonance imagery

(MRI) test. The MRI is a high-tech, state-of-the-art machine that provides a clear picture, not only of the spinal bones, but also the discs and surrounding soft tissues such as muscles, ligaments, and nerves. The essential information the MRI provided in Jimmy's case was the fact that there was no herniated spinal disc. In many cases where a disc has severely herniated, there is no good alternative to the neurosurgeon's knife. Fortunately for Jimmy, he was not a candidate for surgery.

The most telling part of Jimmy's chiropractic examination was the marked restriction of movement I felt in the spinal joints of the upper part of his neck. This finding indicated that Jimmy had a vertebral subluxation complex, in which restricted movement of the vertebrae causes abnormal nerve signaling. This, in turn, can bring about pain, muscle tension, and various other problems. In Jimmy's case, the situation had had two decades to take hold.

But there was more to Jimmy's problem than the fixated vertebrae. Many headaches are caused by vertebral problems in the neck, but it's also important to search out other contributing factors, since both nutrition and emotions can play significant roles. When I asked about his dietary habits, the expression on Jimmy's face told me immediately that he knew himself to be something less than a model citizen in this area. The diet he described was virtually devoid of greenery and whole grains, but suffered no shortages when it came to pork chops, cube steak, coffee, and cola drinks. He also smoked two packs of cigarettes a day, which was an improvement over what until recently had been a four-pack-a-day habit.

He would often wash down his painkillers, muscle relaxants, and lithium with a large cup of coffee or a sixteen-ounce cola drink, and then top it off with a few cigarettes. Frequently, after a full day's work, wired by this chemical mix, he would stay up nearly the entire night, taking care of business paperwork or playing his guitar.

Jimmy was clearly treading on shaky emotional and physical ground. He presented me with a very challenging case, one in which it seemed his life might even depend on whether we could solve the problem. I felt strongly that Jimmy's treatment would need to be holistic in order for us to have a reasonable chance of success. Surgery was not warranted in his case, and he was already taking the strongest medications available. He had pursued the conventional medical route as far as it could go. Chiropractic adjustments for his neck and upper back would be the central focus of my treatment plan, but I knew our chances for a breakthrough would greatly increase if he would make significant dietary changes and also start learning to relax with meditation.

Though I knew from the start that diet changes and meditation would be needed, I decided to wait a while before asking him to begin them. I have found in the past that if I push patients to make major changes quickly, some feel overwhelmed, which can have the unintended effect of discouraging them from even starting. I would much rather wait awhile until the patient is ready, instead of burning their circuits by downloading all the information to them at once.

I reach these decisions on a completely individual basis, relying on all the intuition I can muster. When our rapport has grown strong enough and I see the opening clearly, I plow right in.

The first spinal manipulation I gave Jimmy was a side-posture adjustment of the top vertebra in his neck, delivered on a table with a drop-mechanism designed specifically for adjusting the upper neck. Unlike some chiropractic adjustments, this one does not result in an audible click or pop when administered. It is rarely uncomfortable, but can be surprising the first time. Therefore, I always take time to explain to the patient what I'm going to do and what it will probably feel like.

When he returned two days later, Jimmy reported that his first headache after our initial visit had felt different in quality, less severe and "more spread out" than previous episodes. By the following visit, he said his neck and shoulder pain were decreasing, which pleased him greatly. His headaches, however, continued to be extremely bothersome. After a week in which his headaches showed mild, gradual improvement, but during which he was still taking large quantities of medication, I decided that our rapport was good enough to talk to him in depth about diet.

Summoning all my persuasive powers, I made my pitch and asked for his help. I was convinced that caffeine, cigarettes, and poor diet would significantly impede his recovery. I suggested that we start with some small-to-medium-sized steps in the right direction.

"I want to suggest that you gradually cut back on the cigarettes and coffee and substitute fruit juice, water, or herbal tea for the soft drinks," I told him. "Let's make these changes step by step. You don't have to feel you've got to do it all at once." I probably repeated two or three times that he was welcome to make the changes at whatever pace felt comfortable to him.

"Do you like almonds, peanuts, or sunflower seeds?" I asked.

"I sure do," he answered.

I knew it would be important to keep Jimmy's blood sugar level from dipping too low, because otherwise the craving for sweets and caffeine might prove overwhelming. The well-balanced vegetable protein and unsaturated fat content of nuts and seeds, eaten in moderation, can help accomplish this.

"O.K., then try taking some of those with you in your truck each day and have a handful whenever you feel a craving for sweets. And make a giant salad for lunch, adding some chicken, tuna, or cheese if you like. A slice or two of whole grain bread would also be fine."

At that same visit, I talked with Jimmy about meditation or "quiet time." I suggested that he close his eyes, breathe calmly, and repeat to himself a calming phrase (mantra) of his own choosing, consistent with his own personal beliefs. He chose the word "peace" for his mantra, and I had him practice it there in the office with me, silently saying "peace" whenever his mind started to wander, bringing it back to center.

After sitting quietly for a while, as Jimmy tested the waters of this unfamiliar mental exercise, I said, "Jimmy, if you are serious about going for the gold, becoming headache-free once and for all, you need to make a serious commitment to follow through on all the changes we've been speaking about." A gradual approach was fine, I explained, as long as he persisted in his commitment.

He said he'd do it, and I wondered if he'd have the willpower.

I need not have underestimated him. He stopped the coffee and cola drinks cold turkey, substituting fruit juice and water for his usual daily intake of twelve to twenty-two cups of coffee and a few sixteen-ounce colas.

Riding a high wave of hope and motivation, he took a big plastic bowl of salad to work every day, ate his sunflower seeds, and cut back his smoking to one pack a day. At home, he ate whole grain cereal for breakfast and plenty of vegetables with his dinner. His wife, who had been trying for years to convince him to eat vegetables, could not have been more pleased with the changes.

Within a few days, Jimmy was able for the first time in years to sleep through the night without interruption and discovered that he needed less medication to keep the pain at an acceptable level. He also reported a feeling of increased strength in his left arm, which no longer hurt as sharply or for as long a time after heavy labor.

As we continued Jimmy's chiropractic adjustments, I found a gradually increasing freedom of movement in the vertebral joints of his neck and upper back. The innate self-healing ability of Jimmy's body, no longer blocked to the same degree by spinal subluxations and nutritional inadequacy, was reawakening from its lengthy slumber.

Jimmy kept up his daily meditation and reported an interesting phenomenon. He found that when he moved into a deepened state of relaxation, he could move the pain from one area of his body to another. Experimenting with this, he moved his neck pain down his arm into his wrist. The next day, he was dismayed to discover that while his neck felt better, his wrist was extremely painful. Jimmy had never experienced this sense of power over his mind and body before and came to me somewhat perplexed.

I explained that mind and body overlap at all levels of our being and that the phenomenon he had happened upon was well known and had, in fact, been researched in depth at places like the Menninger Foundation in Kansas. I told him that the power he had tapped into was altogether natural, an ability shared by us all, and that it was important to use it with respect and care. I suggested that if he wished to experiment with moving the pain around, the next time he should direct it to leave his body alto-gether. Jimmy followed these directions, and though he couldn't fully eliminate his neck pain, he had no further difficulty with his wrist.

We continued his chiropractic adjustments, and Jimmy re-mained true to his commitment, following his new diet and continuing to meditate. After three weeks, his headaches had ceased altogether and he longer required any medication. He stopped smoking entirely and found that when he tried to smoke a few cigarettes on a particularly stressful day, they no longer tasted good.

Jimmy was in treatment with me for one month. By the end of that time, he was free from headaches and had minimal neck and shoulder discomfort. Follow-up a year later confirmed that there had been no return of Jimmy's once-fearsome headaches and that his dependence on prescription medications was a thing of the past.

Had he kept up all the good habits begun while under treat-ment? Yes and no.

"We all have our weaknesses. I go back and forth with smoking. I stop and start, and then stop again. I still eat the salads frequently, and I eat all sorts of vegetables—corn, peas, broccoli. I drink water, lots of it. I drink it off and on all day. I've gotten to the point where I prefer the taste of water over soft drinks. They taste too syrupy, although every once in a while I have to have a Dr. Pepper®. I do have a cup or two of coffee a day. I've got little bags of peanuts in my lunch. I'm very conscious of it. Sometimes I'll eat junk food for a week. Spend a lot of money. Then I stop. I think, what am I doing this for? I feel worse and it costs more!"

* * *

People with twenty-year headaches don't walk into my office every day of the year. But I did have a case my first year in practice, which gave me an initial sense of just how powerful chiropractic and natural healing methods can be in dealing with this problem.

Cheri, a systems analyst for the federal government, was thirty-nine when she came to me. Short and heavy-set, she had been having headaches since high school. For the previous five years, these headaches had occurred on a daily basis. On most days, she would wake up with a headache, but if she was fortunate enough to awaken pain-free, she could count on the pain appearing by 11:00 a.m. Usually, it would peak in intensity around 3:00 in the afternoon. She explained to me how she had come to rely on medication as a daily ritual:

> "Back in the beginning, aspirin would be all I'd need. I'd take one or two of those, and bye-bye headache. It worked like magic. Then the magic started to wear off. It would ease the pain, but wouldn't relieve it completely. So I'd take another dose."

She found herself needing to take more and more medication to achieve the same level of relief:

> "After a while, I went to the doctor. He gave me a prescription, and at first that seemed to work just fine. But after a few months, I started to need more of it. And more, and more. Eventually, I graduated to a stronger medication. I was on a merry-go-round and I couldn't figure out how to get off."

Over the next decade and a half, Cheri required higher and higher doses of stronger and stronger prescription medicines. By the time she came for a chiropractic evaluation, she was taking the maximum allowable dosage of the strongest available prescription medication for migraine headaches. While this medication had previously eased the pain, she had reached the point where it was no longer working. Cheri looked calm on the outside, but she made it clear to me immediately that she was on the edge of desperation.

"If you can even make it so that the medication works again, I'll be eternally grateful," she said. "Anything else is more than I can bring myself to hope for. If you can't, I don't know what I'll do."

It is unfortunately still true that, for many people, a chiropractor is someone to go to only after all else has failed. This was certainly the case with Cheri. For chiropractors, the silver lining behind this cloud comes from the fact that when we are able to help such people, for whom all else has clearly failed, there is no question as to the effectiveness of our methods. Such satisfied patients are the reason chiropractic has spread so far and wide by word of mouth for the past century. More than twenty million Americans now visit a chiropractor each year.

With Cheri, as with all new patients, I took a case history in which I gave her the opportunity to discuss any health issue she thought might be relevant. It turned out that aside from the headaches, she also was experiencing paresthesia (a combination of tingling and numbness) in her hands several times a week. Since the nerves that supply the hands come from the neck, this clue pointed toward a vertebral problem in the neck. She also mentioned that her gall bladder had been removed and that she had had a hysterectomy several years earlier. Following the hysterectomy, she had gained eighty pounds.

Her physical examination was, for the most part, unremarkable. Her reflexes were normal and there was no numbness in her arms or hands when a pinwheel was passed across them. Her blood pressure was moderately elevated at 140/90, but this is at the uppermost end of the normal range, not so high that it could reasonably be considered the cause of her headaches.

I sent her to a medical radiologist for x-rays, to be certain that no tumors or other unexpected disease processes were present. Fortunately, none were. She did have some moderate arthritic changes (thinning of a spinal disc, with small calcium spurs) in the lower neck, but again these were not of sufficient severity to explain her headaches. All in all, there was nothing that would have indicated to a typical medical physician what the source of her problem could be.

But to someone trained as a chiropractor or an osteopath (in the United States, osteopathic training includes the full medical school curriculum, plus courses in manipulative therapy), there were definite telltale clues. First, there was a heightened sensitivity to pressure in the uppermost part of Cheri's neck, just below the skull. Second, and most significantly, there was restricted movement of the joint where the occiput (the large, curved bone in back of the skull) meets the atlas vertebra (the top bone in the neck). While I could not know for certain that the vertebral subluxation at the top of Cheri's neck was the cause of her headaches, my training told me that there was a good chance of a causal connection.

I was explaining all this to her, going over the x-rays and making my recommendations, when a thunderstorm passed through town and blew out all the electricity in the building. This had never happened to me before while I was with a patient, and for a moment I thought I should call it a day and send her home. Then it dawned on me in a warm and comforting flash that, unlike so many other things in our high-tech society, chiropractic did not require electricity. There was enough light coming through the window from outdoors to adequately illumine the room, and my chiropractic table (and my hands) didn't have to be plugged in. The two of us had a good laugh about it, and then I adjusted her atlas vertebra. We set up an appointment for a few days later, and she headed home.

Cheri arrived at her next visit with a strange request.

"Should I kiss your shoes?" she asked, and then started laughing.

At first I was quite taken aback and replied that I didn't think it was such a great idea. I wouldn't be surprised if I turned a medium shade of crimson during this exchange.

"It's definitely working," she explained. "The medicine is working again. And the headaches don't feel the same. It's more like a 'heaviness' than a fullblown headache. It's incredible. Even if it never gets better than this, if it will just stay this good, I thank God for my good fortune."

I told her I was very excited to hear this was happening, but that I hoped it was just the beginning, with better things to come.

"I want to reach a point where you no longer feel a need to use any medicine at all," I said. "It's fine with me if you use it when you feel you have to, but I really believe that if there can be this big a shift so soon, much more progress is possible. I don't know how long it will take, but let's see if we can do it."

"By the way, I was just kidding about kissing your shoes," she said with a smile.

Other changes were also occurring. After the first chiropractic adjustment, Cheri found that her nose started running for an hour or so, at which point it suddenly stopped. After that, she could breathe through both nostrils, something that she had not been able to do for as long as she could remember. Though she hadn't considered this nasal congestion worth mentioning when I took her history, she certainly found its sudden disappearance noteworthy. Within a week, her blood pressure also dropped to 128/90, still not normal, but definitely a step in the right direction. Over the next month, Cheri tapered down her use of medications. There were ups and downs along the way, with a sharp headache occasionally punctuating a relatively comfortable few days. She reached the point where her use of prescription medication became the exception rather than the rule.

Several weeks into treatment, it seemed to me that we were reaching a plateau of sorts. Asked to rate her improvement on a scale of zero to one hundred (with zero being the point where we had started and one hundred meaning there were no more headaches at all), she rated herself at eighty. On the one hand, this was wonderful. On the other, we seemed to be making no further progress.

Cheri remained pleased as punch, however, and kept repeating that even if it never got any better, that was no problem. But by now I had set my sights on complete cessation of all her headaches, and I started considering supplemental approaches. I sent Cheri to a hospital laboratory for a six-hour glucose tolerance test, which determines whether any blood sugar abnormalities are present. A high reading can indicate diabetes, while either a low reading or an unusual pattern of fluctuation can suggest hypoglycemia (low blood sugar).

Cheri's lab results pointed toward low blood sugar, and I recommended appropriate dietary changes. As I would do with
Jimmy a decade later, I had her start eating lots of vegetables,
along with small amounts of protein foods spread throughout
the day. I also asked her to refrain completely from cola drinks
(which on some days she had been having at all three meals),
alcohol, and whatever other junk-food carbohydrates she was
accustomed to.

She stuck to the diet religiously and her headaches soon disappeared entirely. In addition, within a few days after altering her
diet, Cheri's blood pressure dropped to 120/80, smack dab in the
middle of normal range, and it stayed there. Over the next year,
her headaches returned only when she went off her diet, splurg-
ing on some ice cream or a couple of glasses of wine on special
occasions.

"Sometimes I just decide it's worth it," she told me. "I'm willing to have a headache now and then. Knowing that I can stop it
the next day, I don't mind so much."

Cheri came in for a chiropractic adjustment once every few
months for the next two years, at which point she concluded that
she was cured. She referred her father and her roommate to me
for help with their back pain, and the last I heard of her was five
years after our last visit. She sent regards to me through her roommate and let me know that she had been completely free of
headaches for three years.

* * *

Chiropractors are well known for helping people with back
and neck pain, but our success with headaches is a surprise to
many. One of the best, most unbiased reports on this and related
issues was done by a government commission in New Zealand,
which was charged with evaluating the appropriateness of including chiropractic services in their national health insurance
program.[2] After lengthy study, in which they assessed all available evidence pro and con, the initially skeptical commissioners
endorsed chiropractic inclusion in the national system, without

a medical doctor's referral, for back pain, neck pain, and headaches. These are the three areas where the evidence supporting chiropractic is most compelling.

I have seen a great many cases in my practice, as have the other chiropractors I know, where headaches have decreased or vanished in response to chiropractic care, sometimes after years of having been nonresponsive to traditional medical treatment.

I look forward to a time not too far in the future when it will be altogether ordinary for medical physicians to refer their headache patients to chiropractors. I don't want too many more people to wait through twenty years—or even twenty days—of agony.

CHAPTER 3

DOLORES' FULL CIRCLE: A BODY-MIND JOURNEY

Dolores walked slowly into my office, cautiously holding herself to avoid the acute lower back and abdominal pains that any sharp or unexpected movement could bring. A striking olive-skinned woman, she had been referred to me by a massage therapist who saw the need for an in-depth evaluation.

While lower back and abdominal pain were Dolores' most bothersome symptoms when she came to see me, a long and convoluted journey had preceded them. Her original symptoms, more than a decade earlier, had been emotional. A few years after Dolores immigrated to the United States from Latin America, her alcoholic mother, who had stayed behind, committed suicide. Relatives blamed Dolores. From that time on, she was plagued with bouts of depression.

Renowned American neurosurgeon and pain specialist Norman Shealy, M.D., has theorized that most physical illness begins with depression. Dolores certainly provides a case in point:

"I was depressed for many years, sometimes so depressed I could not get out of my bed. Then after a while I would get well and start going strong. I remember one Christmas I planned a party and invited everybody. For that one month I was terrific. It's amazing. I would clean house, move things, and make everything wonderful. Christmas came, and then after it was over I went back into my depression. I would be depressed for two to three weeks, and then get up and try to do something."

While depression begins in the mind and spirit, it can quickly cross into the physical realm, affecting the body as well:

"When I was depressed, I would be sleeping many hours a day. It was unbelievably hard to wake up. Sometimes I would be asleep, but it was as if I were awake—I could hear things in the house, but it became part of a dream. Then I would go into a deep sleep again."

Dolores was the mother of three young children, so she could never get as much rest as she wanted and needed. Her husband was gone at work much of the time, so the daily household and family chores remained her responsibility. At times even simple tasks seemed overwhelming:

"The children went to school, and I had to get them ready. It was such a struggle waking up in the morning. I would have to make breakfast for them, struggling with all my power to stay awake for that hour in the kitchen. As soon as they were out the door, I would immediately go back to sleep. I wouldn't get up until they came home from school. I'd take a shower and cook some dinner, and then by seven o'clock I was asleep for the night."

It was the most difficult period of Dolores' life. At times, she and those around her felt she might be going off the deep end:

"Several times I saw something walking with me. It was

like a shadow, but it was not a shadow. When I walked in the hallway, from one room to another, it would go 'Ah!' and scare me to death. It looked like somebody was there, close to me. But a moment later I would look around and see that nobody but me was in the house, and I would think, 'I'm scared of myself.' "

Dolores went to a psychiatrist, who told her she was hallucinating. Dolores herself was of two minds about this. Part of her accepted the psychiatrist's professional judgment, while another part believed she was seeing spirits. In her native land, such an explanation would have been altogether normal. Here in the United States, it was culturally unacceptable.

Shortly after visiting the psychiatrist, Dolores began to get severe headaches. She was taken to the hospital and thoroughly examined with all the technology modern medicine had to offer. Blood and urine tests, brain scans, and a spinal tap were performed, but none revealed a physical cause for her headaches.

One of the unfortunate paradoxes of medical technology, and of technology in general, is that the advanced methods used to diagnose or treat a problem can sometimes cause other problems. In the health field, ailments resulting from medical intervention are called "iatrogenic." The next stage of Dolores' illness appears to have had an iatrogenic cause.

Within a few days after the spinal tap (a procedure that involves sticking a long needle directly into the spinal column in order to extract spinal fluid for testing purposes), Dolores developed excruciating pain in the area where the needle had been inserted. In Dolores' words, the pain "felt very sharp, sometimes so sharp that it became numb and I could not move my leg."

Interestingly, when the back pain began, the intensity of Dolores' headaches decreased sharply. This offered her little consolation, however, since her overall level of pain was worse than ever. Only the location had changed. The lower back pain was with her for the next seven years:

"I would be in terrible pain for months at a time. Twice

the pains were so bad that I went to the emergency room. One of those times, I was on the floor at home, crawling on my hands and knees, trying to get to the telephone to call my husband. That's how bad it was. It felt like my leg *was not there*. It was terribly frightening. I finally pulled myself up and reached the phone, and he came right home. They carried me to the car . . . I remember being embarrassed that the neighbors would see me."

For years Dolores went from doctor to doctor, searching for the ever-elusive cure. Each doctor offered hope in the form of a new pill. Some of the medications offered temporary relief from the worst of the pain, but none made it go away completely or maintained their effect for very long.

Some had bothersome side effects:

"The doctors gave me medicines—painkillers, muscle relaxants. I was changing from doctor to doctor. After six months or so with a doctor, I would realize he wasn't going to help me and that he really didn't know what was wrong with me. None of them knew. The pains would still be there just as bad afterward as they were before."

Because they were not trained to do so, none of the physicians had examined Dolores' spine the way a chiropractor does. If they had, it would have been clear to them immediately that she needed manipulation of her sacroiliac joints and her upper neck. Not until she came to my office, after seven years of often maddening pain, did she have an examination which determined the nature of her problem.

When I examined Dolores, the most unmistakable finding was spasm throughout the muscles of her lower back. I've treated thousands of patients, at least half of them for lower back pain, but I have almost never come across the degree of rigidity I felt in Dolores' lower back that day. I knew immediately why the massage therapist had sent her my way. Her lower back was like a sheet of barely flexible plastic.

When spasm like this occurs, it is not just a case of body mechanisms going haywire. The muscles tense up for a good reason—as a guarding response, to stabilize the area and thereby prevent even worse pain and suffering. The spasm is the body's best way of dealing with a difficult situation. In seeking a solution, the most relevant question for the doctor should not be, "How can I get these muscles to relax?" but rather, "What is causing them to go into spasm? What are they trying to protect her from?"

This is what distinguishes the chiropractic approach to back problems from that of all but the most enlightened medical physicians. The medical approach, in general, is to offer muscle relaxant, anti-inflammatory, and pain-relieving medications to quell the muscle spasm and ease the discomfort. The chiropractor, in contrast, aims to go to a deeper level of causation, correcting the factors that cause the spasm in the first place.

Recent scientific research has demonstrated that spinal manipulation is significantly more effective than the prevalent "bed-rest-plus-medication" approach which is still, unfortunately, the treatment offered by many general practitioners—the physicians who see the largest number of back pain patients. Not only that— recent studies have shown that no treatment at all (the "grin-and-bear-it" approach) even outperforms bed rest and anti-inflammatory medication.[1] Dolores didn't need scientific studies to tell her this. She learned it the old-fashioned way, by following medical advice and reaching a dead end.

As I examined Dolores, I found that when I applied light pressure to certain areas of her lower back and buttocks, the muscles across a wide area jerked involuntarily with pain. This was also true in the right upper portion of her abdomen, in the area of the liver. Her upper neck was also extremely sensitive. I checked her entire spine for areas of restricted joint motion and found parts of her lower back and neck where substantial fixation was present. This indicated a problem more serious than the muscle tension. Often, when subluxations (fixations with nerve irritation) exist, they cause muscle tension.

Fortunately, none of the tests I performed indicated that she had a herniated spinal disc. The tests which determine this are an important part of the initial chiropractic examination, because while chiropractic is helpful for many disc cases, some of the more severe ones need to be referred to a surgeon. A herniated disc can only be definitively diagnosed with a CT scan (a computer-enhanced multilayered x-ray) or an MRI, but physical findings in a normal office examination will, in the vast majority of cases, indicate whether a disc problem is a likelihood.

While it was apparent to me that her lower back required chiropractic adjustments, I was concerned that the muscle tension and sensitivity in that area were so severe that the more dramatic moves in my chiropractic repertoire might prove very uncomfortable.

I have always felt it important to use methods that put the patient at ease whenever possible, so I began our first treatment by utilizing a technique that does not include a thrusting manipulation. I placed padded wedge-like blocks at specific angles under her pelvic bones, which allowed her body's own weight to shift the balance between the two sides of the pelvis. While she was resting on the blocks, I applied a mild, low-volt electrical stimulation to the muscles of the lower back.

Dolores told me later that she felt a mild sense of relief from the blocks alone, but that when the electrical stimulation went on, she for the first time realized that she was going to get well. I rounded out the day's treatment with an adjustment of her contracted left psoas muscle, deep in the abdomen, and some gentle relaxing techniques that are part of polarity therapy.

Before she left the office that first day, I spoke to her about diet and the fact that hers contained no high-fiber foods at all. I explained the importance of fiber and predicted that if she started eating high-fiber foods like whole grains in sufficient amounts, her severe constipation of ten years' duration would probably soon be a thing of the past. I also suggested that her digestive discomfort would likely disappear along with it.

Both of these predictions came true within the first week. Furthermore, acting on a suggestion from the massage therapist who had referred her to me, Dolores applied castor oil packs to her abdomen and lower back and had a colonic irrigation to cleanse her lower bowel.

The castor oil packs particularly impressed her:

> "When I put on the oil, it was as if the pain in the right side of my abdomen just started to melt away. I have never felt anything like it. It was like magic."

The external use of castor oil, often recommended in the Edgar Cayce readings, struck a particularly resonant chord for Dolores:

> "In Trinidad, the last place we lived before coming to the United States, my daughter had a growth on her eye, a bump in the corner of her eye, which was getting bigger. I was very afraid to go to the doctor, because I believe more in the natural healing, the use of herbs. I was afraid they would cut her, and she would lose her eye.
>
> "Castor oil is very famous in my country, and I had some which I had brought with me. I put the oil on a little piece of material, and then I put it on her eye. She slept with that. The growth was gone within a couple of days. I forgot all about this for years. When I came to the United States, I didn't even know the word in English for castor oil. But then, when I came to Virginia Beach and talked to people at the Edgar Cayce Center, it all came back to me. It's the same thing we have at home."

When Dolores returned to my office two days later for her second visit, changes were immediately apparent. She walked without hesitation, and the pained expression on her face was replaced by a radiant smile. She told me that her low back pain had decreased dramatically and that she had been able to arise in the morning with her leg feeling normal for the first time in many months.

When I checked her lower back, little of the muscle spasm remained. The movement of her right sacroiliac joint was completely restored to normal, although the one on the left was still restricted. Dolores said that what remained of her lower back pain was now focused on the left side. I adjusted the restricted left sacroiliac joint, and by the next visit she reported that only a little lower back pain remained. It was, she said, "like a miracle." Similarly, the pain in the area of the liver was ninety percent gone.

Dolores had a regularly scheduled visit with her medical physician later that day and told him with great enthusiasm of her breakthrough. He had been treating her for two years, performing various diagnostic tests and prescribing pain relief medication. She expected him to share in her happiness.

He didn't. He told her she was crazy to go to a chiropractor, loudly proclaiming that "chiropractors can't help anything." When she mentioned that I had theorized that the right upper abdominal pain (now finally gone after being present for years) may have been related to her liver, he said this was "nonsense." He then briefly examined her abdomen, declared that she had a hernia, and recommended immediate surgery. She said, "No, thank you!" and left his office, somewhat shaken but wiser for the experience.

Within two weeks of beginning chiropractic treatment, after just six visits, Dolores was completely free of symptoms. She came in and said to me, "Doctor, I don't think I need to see you any more."

Because I have seen many cases where the symptoms leave before the cause has been fully resolved, I suggested that we schedule one or two more visits, with several days between, to allow me to evaluate whether her spinal condition was indeed stabilized. In addition, I wanted to use those visits to do some additional polarity therapy, which I find to be an excellent balancing technique, a nice finishing touch.

It turned out that Dolores was right—she was fine and stayed that way. Follow-up a year later confirmed that the pains had never returned. In addition, her digestion and bowel regularity remained normal, and she described her outlook on life as more positive than ever before.

Dolores' case raises a number of issues worth examining more deeply. First, there is the question of psychosomatic illness, a complex and multifaceted topic if ever there was one.

Without question, Dolores' initial symptoms were psychological. She was shaken to the core by her mother's suicide and by the subsequent attempts on the part of her relatives to blame her for her mother's death. Her depression was serious and lasted for years. Soon after being told by the psychiatrist that things which seemed real to her (the wraithlike visions she saw in the hallway) were actually imaginary, she developed severe headaches. This turn of events led her doctors to perform the spinal tap, which was followed shortly thereafter by the lower back pain which persisted for seven years until she came to me.

Those are the facts. But what do they mean? What conclusions can we reasonably draw from them? What does Dolores' case tell us about the relationship between body and mind? For one thing, it reminds us that when someone is emotionally upset at a deep level, that individual can create physical symptoms to complement his or her mental state. Since the time of Freud, this idea has become widely accepted. Today it is hardly controversial.

But then the plot thickens. The physical aspect of the ailment takes on a life of its own, affecting the nervous, muscular, and circulatory systems of the body, which undergo very real changes. Nerves transmit electrical messages of pain and irritation, muscles tighten and stay that way, and blood vessels contract and expand in abnormal fashion, depriving some areas of adequate blood supply and oversupplying others. These physical events, in turn, feed back to the patient's conscious awareness, further aggravating the condition. The knot tightens.

In Dolores' case, once the spinal tap was performed, a new level of purely physical causation was superimposed on the already existing psychosomatic problems, complicating them substantially. I think that was the point at which the possibility of solving her case with purely psychological methods ended. Injury had now been added to insult, forming a symptom complex unresponsive to methods which did not treat body and mind together.

So how can chiropractors address body and mind together? First, we must help the body. This is expected of us, focused as our training and practice are on the physical aspects of healing.

As a chiropractor, I look first to the spine, adjusting any subluxations I find and attending to other imbalances of the
muscular system with hands-on methods, supplemented when
necessary by electrical therapies.

But in a case where the mental component is strong, physical
healing methods may fall short, since underlying emotional tension tends to reassert itself at every opportunity. This brings the
swift, insistent return of those physical tensions and restrictions
we have sought to contain or disperse with physical methods.

How then to uncouple the deadly duo of physical and emotional tension? The specifics vary from case to case, but common
themes are present and consistent guidelines emerge. Above all,
it is essential to convey to the patient a sincere belief that healing
is possible. The doctor's positive attitude, both spoken and un-
spoken, is essential in creating or confirming the patient's own
belief that healing can and will occur.

When I spoke with Dolores a year after she completed her
treatment, she gave this point great emphasis:

"When I saw you, you helped me a lot with your positive
attitude. That helped tremendously. When I left here, I said,
'Boy, he's so positive, I better be positive.' Then I got a better
attitude."

I should add that Dolores did more than just decide to change
her attitude. She started to do volunteer work and decided to go
back to school. She put her beliefs into practice.

Hyperbole and grandiose promises by the doctor are not necessary, just a straightforward expression of confidence that the
future need not mirror the worst aspects of the past. Doctors cannot fake this and it is very important that they not try to. Lying or
exaggerating sends a subliminal message contradicting whatever
words are spoken, thereby subtly undercutting the trust between
doctor and patient that must be present for healing to proceed. If
the doctor is unsure, he or she should be truthful about it.

With each patient, when I estimate the length of treatment I
expect he or she will need, I take care to mention that this is based

on the average recovery time in similar cases and that *the client is welcome to exceed the average by as much as possible*. No doctor ever knows in advance the exact course of any patient's healing process, and, while this uncertainty can be a source of fear, it can also serve as an inspiring reminder that we all possess healing capacities far beyond those we have ever needed to call upon. The glass is half full unless we choose to see it as half empty.

*   *   *

Trusting relationships between doctor and patient grow best in an atmosphere of mutual purpose and shared responsibility. While a certain imbalance of power is implicit in any situation where one person is the expert and the other is seeking the expert's help, success in the healing endeavor depends on moving as close to equality as humanly possible.

B. Lewis Barnett, Jr., M.D., Chairman of the Department of Family Medicine at the University of Virginia School of Medicine, makes this point clearly and beautifully in his book *Between the Lines:*

> "The magic moment when both get into the boat and grab one oar apiece—being careful not to let either take both oars—can make all the difference. Why is it that some physicians seem to get better results than others? Could it have something to do with this nick of time I'm trying to address? Two people, seated together, trying to make a decision concerning the welfare and benefit of the patient is an awesome event. It can be the most important and significant decision of that particular person's life—that moment when there is a reaching toward each other . . .
>
> "We are here to work together. We are here to learn how to solve this problem. *We are here, not to be overwhelmed, but to conquer.* We are here to hope. This space allows for silence, if need be, or when words make very little sense. This space allows for tears, for laughter, for long handshakes."[2]

Mutuality of this sort requires a reworking of the doctor-patient relationship, changing the focus from control to partnership. It requires the doctor to be fully open to insight and input from the patient and demands in return that the patient let go of passivity.

The doctor relinquishes power, and the patient relinquishes powerlessness. Each moves away from the comfort of familiar roles toward a new and potentially liberating framework, democratic in essence. No one is in charge. We create the future together. What could be more strengthening to the inner core of the patient than this unexpected acknowledgment of the need for his or her own wholly engaged participation?

I find that putting all of this into words seems an invasion of an intimate space. It's almost like trying to explain how to love someone. No words can ever do it full justice, yet to evade the subject serves only to perpetuate the old patterns.

Patients who seize this opportunity to be full participants in their healing process are the ones likely to achieve the fullest measure of healing. It's like everything else in life—God helps those who help themselves. For the doctors whose goals for their patients include not only healing but empowerment, patients who assume this active role as co-creators of their own health are by far the most satisfying to work with. They may have more questions than others, and they may frequently force the doctor to stretch his or her current level of skill. They aren't less challenging, but they are unquestionably the model to strive for, the gold standard for the creation of the doctor-patient relationship of the future.

CHAPTER 4

LOWER BACK PAIN
AND MORE

For eighteen years after an automobile accident, Robert, a hardware salesman, experienced on-and-off lower back pain. Then, the year before he came to see me, he spent two weeks in the hospital, having lost the ability to urinate and move his bowels due to an acute spinal inflammation called transverse myelitis. Even after he was released from the hospital, a partial numbness from the transverse myelitis remained, causing significantly decreased sensation in his sexual area.

Robert came to me for help with his lower back pain. He assumed that the pelvic numbness was going to be with him forever and considered himself lucky that his illness hadn't left him paralyzed. In fact, he didn't even mention the numbness on his new patient information form, focusing instead on the lower back pain, which was causing him frequent difficulty at work and at home. He was particularly concerned that it might soon prevent him from performing essential job duties, like lifting heavy boxes.

At our first visit, Robert explained what had happened in the automobile accident eighteen years earlier:

> "I was a passenger in a van going down Main Street when a truck unexpectedly darted out of a side street. A bus was blocking the truck driver's view, so he couldn't see us coming. He hit the van, and it spun around. I wasn't wearing a seatbelt, and the force threw me out the door onto the pavement, landing me on my butt. My lower back and buttocks were hit the hardest.
>
> "I got up and walked around, and I felt some discomfort, but I was also in a state of shock. I think for most people in a situation like that, unless you're really incapacitated, you don't fully feel what's going on with your body.
>
> "It wasn't until later that afternoon that I started having pain, along with stiffness and soreness. I saw my family doctor, and after several visits without much change, he said I should go to a chiropractor. I started seeing one, and after several weeks of treatment, I felt fine. I got a lot of relief from the adjustments and had no more problem until the following year."

Lower back pain is regrettably famous for its repeat performances. For many people who incur lower back injuries, the initial episode is just the beginning. Robert was one of these:

> "There was no more problem until over a year later, when I was moving a seventy-five-pound box. I put it on a loading dock and then bent over. When I tried to straighten up, I felt this awful pain in my lower back. I started seeing another chiropractor, who unfortunately didn't do me any good, and then I started seeing an osteopath, who did."

The pain was controlled but chronic, and Robert learned to live with it:

> "I had resigned myself to the idea that my back was never going to get all better. I minimized the pain by doing things

like sleeping on a hard bed, not lifting things that were too heavy, and seeing the osteopath about once a month."

Chronic back pain can have many causes and frequently results from a combination of factors. Muscles and ligaments can be damaged by trauma, stretching past their normal ranges of motion, tearing slightly. These small tears, which the body heals internally with fibrous scar tissue, can prove a source of difficulty later on. They can cause muscles to become undesirably tight and to develop focal points of tension called "trigger points." Sometimes muscles which have been subjected to trauma actually shorten in response, creating stressful imbalances which force other muscles to move in unaccustomed ways or to take on more than their normal workload.

When ligaments (soft-tissue structures that connect one bone to another) are stretched too far, they can permit a joint (a place where two bones meet) to become hypermobile (too loose), a problem diagnosed by gently moving the joint back and forth, thereby eliciting a repeated click. Hypermobile areas are more difficult to deal with than joint fixations (areas of decreased joint movement), because while manipulation can release a joint fixation, it can aggravate a hypermobile area, causing it to become even looser.

Some hypermobile joints respond well to external applications of salt mixed with apple cider vinegar, gradually tightening in response. This seems to work best with small joints close to the surface, like the wrist, ankle, and jaw joints. Unfortunately, this method often proves inadequate. Most cases of joint hypermobility must be treated indirectly, by strengthening and toning nearby muscles, and giving adjustments to restore normal motion in nearby joints that have become fixated to compensate for the loose joint.

Trigger points in muscles, unlike hypermobile joints, are more readily responsive to hands-on therapy. Chiropractors and massage therapists treat trigger points by the application of firm, deep manual pressure. The goal is to override the reflex arc between the spine and the muscle, by which electrical messages are sent to the muscle, instructing it to maintain abnormally high tension.

Janet Travell, M.D., who was President John Kennedy's physician, is the widely respected developer of trigger point theory and practice and the author of the most widely utilized texts on the subject. She recommends a variety of methods, including the "spray and stretch" technique, in which the muscle is covered with an anesthetic spray, stretched while numb, and then warmed with hot packs afterward.

When Robert came to see me, eighteen years after his automobile accident and one year after his hospitalization, he had trigger points in his lower back and buttocks and in his upper neck as well. In addition, there were spinal fixations in the neck and upper back.

The most dramatic finding, however, was the nearly total lack of normal left sacroiliac (SI) joint motion. I checked this with a method called motion palpation, which for the SI joint involves having the patient stand upright, with one hand holding a doorknob or stabilizing bar. With one of my thumbs on the sacrum (the large bone at the bottom of the spine), and the other on the ilium (the upper portion of the pelvic bone), I asked Robert to raise his legs one at a time, bringing his knee toward his chest, as far as it could comfortably go.

I then monitored whether my thumbs were moving up and down along with the movement of his legs. The movement was present when Robert raised his right leg, but not his left. This meant that the left SI joint was fixated and that I should adjust it accordingly. There are several methods I use to adjust the SI. The most common, widely utilized by both chiropractors and osteopaths, involves placing the patient in a side-lying position, with the upper leg flexed toward the chest. I apply a thrusting pressure to the SI with one hand, while stabilizing the patient's shoulder with the other. I use this method often and find it quite effective.

In Robert's case, though, I knew that a local osteopath, a doctor well respected in our community, had already used this method, with mixed results. I, therefore, chose to go another route.

Robert recalls:

"I remember that you did things that my previous chiropractor and osteopath hadn't done before. They pretty
much used a similar repertory of adjustments, but you did
things differently. One is the test where I hold the
doorhandle and I raise my legs separately, and you look at
my hips. Then you used the spring-loaded adjustment of
my lower back. No one had ever done that before. Likewise
with the blocks."

The "spring-loaded adjustment" Robert referred to is part of
the Thompson technique, named after Dr. Clay Thompson, an
Iowa chiropractor with whom I studied when he was in his sev-
enties. This slight-of-frame chiropractor invented an adjusting
table with spring-loaded drop-pieces to enable him to adequately serve some of his more hefty patients. Brilliant in design,
the table in its mechanism offers an excellent alternative (or primary) method of adjusting patients of all shapes and sizes.

The "blocks" were the brainchild of Dr. Major deJarnette, a
Nebraska chiropractor. These are padded wedges which are
placed at specific angles under the pelvic bones. Like the drop-
piece mechanism, they also grew out of a need for alternative
methods for managing lower back cases, when the traditional
side-posture adjustment was either unsuccessful or contraindicated.

I used both the drop-piece and the blocks at Robert's first visit.
The results were promising. When he returned two days later, his
lower back was feeling much more comfortable. He felt a bit off
balance with certain body movements, but also felt a major shift
was taking place. In addition, when he went home after his first
adjustment, his bowels evacuated fully for the first time in recent
memory.

I saw Robert every other day for the first couple of weeks. By
the third visit, he was able to painlessly turn around in his car to
look at the traffic behind him, something he had been unable to
do for several years. I told him we were clearly on the right track
and gave him some exercises to help stabilize his lower back.

I suggested he start with a commonly prescribed exercise, the
knee-chest stretch (see Figure 11, page 184), in which he would

lie on his back, bend his leg at the knee, and then pull the knee up toward his chest. This would be done first with the left leg, then the right, and then both together. In addition, I had him begin practicing a yoga posture where he would sit cross-legged and bend forward, reaching a point of equilibrium and staying there for a full minute or two, followed by much briefer (five seconds each) bends at a forty-five-degree angle, to the right and then to the left.

At our fourth visit, a week after we had begun, Robert told me, "I feel the best I've felt in years. My whole lower back is looser, more flexible and less painful." Two other changes had also occurred, the proverbial good news and bad news.

I asked for the bad news first. He told me he was experiencing a return of his chronic constipation. This was my cue to speak with him about nutrition. His diet was generally consistent with what I normally recommend, but somewhat low on dietary fiber. I suggested that he eat more whole grain cereals, and this, along with his decision to start eating prunes, resulted in a long-term solution.

The good news that day, which was unquestionably the lead story, was that *full sensation had returned to his groin area.* After having been half-numb for the year since his release from the hospital, his sexual organs felt normal again.

"During the year after the hospitalization, my sexual feelings weren't as they used to be. Urination was fine and defecation was fine, if somewhat irregular. For that I was grateful. But I noticed that I had trouble getting and sustaining an erection and also that my scrotum was partially numb. It had only about half as much feeling as it used to.

"It returned to normal shortly after you started treating me. I hadn't even thought about it. I just suddenly realized that the numbness was gone. It shocked and delighted me. I had thought, 'Well, this is it. This is a legacy of the transverse myelitis, and I've just got to deal with it for the rest of my life.' Well, it isn't!"

Sexual dysfunction has many causes, some emotional and some physical. Among the physical causes, hormonal imbal-

ances and failure of proper nerve transmission figure prominently. Chiropractic adjustments, by unblocking the electrical
flow in the nerves that course from the spine to the organs, can
bring about a cure in some of the cases where the cause lies
within the nervous system. This certainly appears to have happened in Robert's case.

There are as yet no scientific studies proving the efficacy of
chiropractic in cases of pelvic numbness and sexual dysfunction.
The evidence thus far is anecdotal, composed of case studies of
people like Robert. Chiropractic research priorities have for the
most part been directed to those areas—lower back pain, neck
pain, and headaches—which comprise the lion's share of
chiropractic patient populations. It is hoped that, as the scientific validation of these primary conditions is completed over the
next decade (see Chapter Eight), full-fledged studies on cases like
sexual dysfunction, dysmenorrhea (painful menstruation), and
other internal organ problems amenable to chiropractic care will
become far more common.

Over the next several months of Robert's treatment, I gradually decreased his frequency of visits and added to his exercise
regimen. He was a dedicated, cooperative partner in this endeavor, and his progress exceeded my expectations. Sometimes,
after a particularly demanding day at work, his lower back would
act up, but it took more and more to trigger this reaction. Corre-
spondingly, with each episode, less treatment was needed to
bring him back to normal. He recalled three years later:

> "At the beginning, we had to see each other fairly often,
> maybe two or three times a week, but after a while we
> reached a point where even if I threw my back out at work,
> it wouldn't take that long to get it back to normal. Instead of
> requiring weeks like it used to, it might be a couple of visits.
> The very worst has been three, and it's rarely more than one."

One key to the long-lasting nature of Robert's recovery was
that he took an active role in recovering and maintaining his
health:

"I've started doing yoga again. That seems to help a lot, because I'm a lot more relaxed, much looser. I do it once a week, at a class. Then I do various yoga exercises at home when I feel the need, especially when I need to loosen up my lower back or my neck and shoulders. I do it so much that I almost do it spontaneously now."

Aside from the stretching postures he learned in yoga class, Robert started swimming and going bicycle riding. He even took up rollerblading. He didn't tell me about the rollerblading until he had already been at it for a few months. Had he told me earlier, I might well have sounded a strongly cautionary note, for fear that he might injure himself.

But sometimes my patients teach me a thing or two. Robert convinced me that rollerblading was good for him. It's something he loves, and if you find exercise enjoyable, you're more likely to do it regularly and to relax with it. Once Robert knew his body could handle rollerblading, he had the confidence to start working out with weights at the gym. While he initially felt concerned that he would use too much weight and hurt his back, he found that as long as he was careful, the weightlifting caused no problems other than occasional mild soreness.

These days, I see Robert once every few months, if he feels his back is out of adjustment or just in need of a general tune-up. He is living proof that not all chronic problems need be permanently disabling.

*   *   *

Joseph was a thirty-two-year-old association executive in downtown Washington, D.C., where the number of stressed-out executives, lawyers, and government workers approaches epidemic proportions. Typical for the town, Joseph worked very long hours, and his body was paying the price. Formerly a cross-country runner, he was now forty pounds overweight. His middle and lower back hurt almost all the time, and the pain often radiated around to his abdomen on the right side.

His medical physician had diagnosed this as "radiculitis," meaning pain resulting from pressure on a spinal nerve root. When a nerve root is irritated in this way, it can cause pain in that part of the back and can also adversely affect the function of organs supplied by that nerve. Joseph experienced frequent discomfort in his lower abdomen and groin, especially when urinating, and his urologist considered this a result of the radiculitis. It was frequently accompanied by a low-grade fever.

He was not a happy camper when we first met. "I really need help with this, and I hope you're the one who can do it," he told me when we sat down in the consultation room. "It's driving me up a wall."

Then he shared his variation of a story I had heard many times before of a seemingly endless series of time-consuming and expensive tests, which had, when all was said and done, told him a great deal about the problems he didn't have, but precious little about those he did have:

> "Doc, I'm in pain most of the time, but even more than that, I'm bone-tired. I'm tired, but I can't sleep. I know I need seven or eight hours of sleep a night, but I hardly ever get more than four or five. I'm taking a prescription medication to help me sleep, but it leaves me drowsy in the morning, and it doesn't let me get enough sleep anyway. I started out on a different medicine, but that was even worse—way too strong."

He described going through test after test, none of which seemed to show anything wrong:

> "I've had an upper GI and a lower GI series (x-rays of the digestive tract), and I've had ultrasound and CT-scans of my abdomen. The long and short of it is, I'm no better off than when I started. I know that I don't have a tumor or an ulcer, but nothing they've been able to find out has done a darn thing to make me any better. It's frustrating and it's tiring.
> "I've tried with all my might to figure out what's causing

this back pain. As far as I can tell, my poor posture sure doesn't help, and my job involves long periods where I just sit all day. I know those are contributing to my problems, but I'm hoping you can find something else, something that lets you know what to do to help. I've heard good things about chiropractors for years, and I've finally decided to give one of you guys a try."

Joseph mentioned on his new patient form that both of his parents were legally disabled; his father from back pain due to an old army injury and his mother from severe bursitis and calcium deposits in her back. He didn't come right out and say it, but I sensed that Joseph was worried that he was heading down the same path. It's not an unreasonable fear; some back disorders do have a hereditary component. I told Joseph that I would do my best to help him and that I wanted it to be a team effort. Somewhere not too far down the line, I said, I would probably be asking him to put some extra effort into what we both hoped would be a process of recovery.

When I first examined Joseph, the most obvious problem was that when he stood up straight, hands at his sides, his right hip was clearly lower than his left. A small amount of asymmetry is usually not a big problem, but this was more than a small amount. As I expected, there was significant sensitivity when I pressed certain areas in his middle and lower back. Some movements, such as one called Kemp's Test, where the patient is bent back and to the side, brought increased lower back pain. Other than that, however, there were no red flags in sight. I took x-rays of Joseph's lower spine and pelvis with him standing up. X-rays taken in the upright, weight-bearing posture provide information helpful in determining how much a short leg, if present, is affecting someone's pelvic and lower back balance. That way the effects of gravity are taken into account, and the doctor can reach an informed judgment as to whether a heel lift should be inserted into the patient's shoe on the short leg side.

Joseph's films showed a clear pelvic tilt. Taking various factors into account, I was able to determine that his right leg was approximately twenty-six millimeters (about an inch) shorter than his left, among the largest leg length disparities I have seen. Rather than immediately putting in a lift, I first wanted to see how significant a change we could achieve with adjustments alone. I explained to Joseph that within a month or so, we would start with a small lift and gradually increase its height until we reached the proper level.

Sometimes, if too large a lift is inserted right away, this can cause a sharp increase in lower back pain, as the back muscles are forced abruptly to stretch or contract in unaccustomed ways. Joseph readily agreed that he would just as soon avoid that. At that same first visit, I adjusted his right sacroiliac joint with the drop-piece technique, and I also had him rest for several minutes on the pelvic blocks.

Within two visits, Joseph felt no pain on the left side of his back, and the pain on the right had substantially decreased in intensity. He drove to Georgia to visit his parents for Thanksgiving and found that his back hurt far less than it had on similar trips the past few years. When he felt his lower back starting to tighten up on some of the long stretches rolling down the interstate, he followed a travel suggestion of mine. He pulled off at a rest stop and rolled down the window. Then, standing outside the car, he gripped his hands over the bottom of the open window, stabilizing himself, and then leaned back into a squatting position for a minute or so, stretching out those tight lower back muscles.

On his return, Joseph had more surprising news for me. He was sleeping like a baby at night, without any medication. On the vacation, he had slept nine to ten hours a night, and now he was even able to get eight hours of sleep a night during a hectic workweek. This was a dramatic change for the better. He was able to relax, despite the unchanged demands of a job where seventy hours a week was considered par for the course.

As excited as I was to hear this good news, there was more. His problems with urination had disappeared. The stream was normal, the pain was gone, and so was the fever. Like Robert, he had come seeking treatment for lower back pain and discovered to his surprise that chiropractic is capable of helping more than bad backs. The urinary pain and dysfunction never returned in the three years I worked with Joseph before I moved from Washington to Virginia Beach.

Buoyed by the improvement in his back pain, Joseph increased his exercise activity, going to the gym more frequently and working out more vigorously. It had been more than two years since this former star athlete had been able to let loose physically like this and he was ecstatic.

"It was like a tremendous weight being lifted off my shoulders. I could use my body like an athlete again. All through the time I was growing up, I would work off stress with physical activity. I would run for miles, and I never felt freer. Then, when my back went bad and I developed the radiculitis, I always had to hold back, for fear that I would end up on my back for days or weeks. Now, for the first time in years, I can go all out again. What a pleasure!"

As planned, I put a small (five-millimeter) lift into Joseph's right shoe after a month of treatment. He did experience some lower back discomfort from it, but that was just a transitional phase, and within a few days it felt normal again. Soon he found that he could walk farther without fatigue. Over the next few months, we gradually worked our way up to a half-inch lift, and this seemed to provide adequate support. Joseph felt that he was walking straighter, and his back pain stayed well controlled. On occasion, when his stress level was highest and he had to cut back on his exercise, he would come in complaining of increased pain. But these episodes became increasingly rare, and eventually we saw each other only once every month or two.

Joseph mentioned to me once, several months after we started treatment, that he had left the heel lift out of his shoe for a few days, and the radicular pain had returned. He truly needed it to maintain proper spinal balance, and, realizing this, he made certain to have one in each set of shoes from that point onward. Since Joseph's lower back had felt so well prior to using the lift, it may seem strange that removing it for a short time would result in such discomfort.

The explanation is that while bodies have great powers of adaptation, they sometimes respond poorly to mixed messages or fast changes. Once a heel lift has been inserted, the body adapts to the altered biomechanics. Taking away the lift forces it to adapt once again, and that adaptation can mean increased tension in certain muscles and joints and hence renewed back pain.

The next spring, when the pink cherry blossoms and fragrant blooming magnolias were gracing Washington with the peak of their beauty, Joseph came in burdened with a full-blown case of hayfever. He asked if there was anything I could do to help.

I used to be a hayfever sufferer myself and still have some tendencies in that direction, so I really empathize when someone comes in sniffling and red-eyed. I remember times as a child and a young adult when my consciousness seemed to be located about half an inch behind my nose for months on end. While this was happening, my mind felt clouded, and I found it a real effort to relate to people. I also faced a constant unpleasant choice between antihistamines and a runny nose. So when Joseph came in stuffed up and sniffly, I knew what he was going through.

During the many springs and summers when my ability to enjoy life seemed to rise and fall with the pollen count, I had the opportunity to sample all sorts of remedies, conventional and unconventional. As a youngster, I used the usual prescription and over-the-counter medications with mixed success. Later, I tried many approaches I read about in books; at various times I did things like eliminating dairy from my diet for months, cutting out all processed foods, eating a mostly raw-food diet, taking high doses of vitamin and mineral supplements, and more.

None of these worked that well for me. Then in 1979 I came across the book, *Body, Mind, and Sugar*, written in the 1950s by E.M. Abrahamson, M.D. Based on his own clinical research, Abrahamson concluded that there was a direct correlation among allergies, asthma, and low blood sugar, which could be remedied by adhering to a diet specifically designed to balance blood sugar levels.

I read this book when I was a chiropractic student. It was June in Iowa, and the pollen count was astronomical. I had been ex-

periencing severe hayfever symptoms for a month and was desperate for relief. But at the same time, I did not want to merely
suppress the symptoms with medication. I decided that if Dr.
Abrahamson's claims were even half true, following his advice
would be worth a try. I went on his diet, and *within a day all my
symptoms were gone.* The pollen count continued to hover
around 250, but my body no longer found that to be a problem.
As you can imagine, this experience had a strong effect on me.

In its original form, Abrahamson's diet, which at the time was
the standard medical diet for low blood sugar, has some real
drawbacks. Its fat and protein content is higher than what we
now know is healthy for the cardiovascular system. It also sharply
limits intake of carbohydrates, even good ones like whole grains
and fruits. The diet includes frequent small meals throughout the
day, with protein foods like meat, cheese, nuts, and seeds featured prominently and permits an unlimited amount of almost
all vegetables.

Personally, I stayed on it rigorously for a few months and then
started to branch out. Eventually, I was able to change over to a
largely vegetarian diet without my allergies acting up. I believe
that the Abrahamson diet strengthened me to the point where I
no longer needed it. I now use a modified version of the
Abrahamson approach (much lower in fat and protein, with
more whole grains) occasionally, when the need arises.

Joseph not only lost his allergies on the modified Abrahamson
diet—over the next four months, he also lost forty-one pounds.
He would update me periodically about his visits to the tailor,
who was apparently having trouble keeping up with Joseph's fast-
shrinking waistline.

The overweight, overburdened, aging Washington white-col-
lar worker with chronic lower back pain had metamorphosed
into a slender, mostly pain-free young man. Within the next year,
he left his job to accept an offer from a smaller company, which
paid him the same salary and offered a much saner schedule.

Chapter 5

Angela and the Road Not Taken

The most dramatic stories of recovery come from people whose problems were so severe that recovery seemed impossible. Angela's story is among the most dramatic I've seen. More than once, she came back from the edge of death, surviving by dint of her own intelligence and daring, along with a strong dollop of what I can only call the grace of God.

Angela was fifty when she came to me as a patient, and the history of her past physical challenges could fill a spellbinding book. The story begins when, after a basically normal and healthy childhood, Angela fell on her back at school when she was a thirteen-year-old eighth grader in Pittsburgh.

"I had a very bad fall. I fell backward. We had these wooden desks at school with seats you could raise up and down. They had frames with wrought ironwork. When I fell, my seat happened to be up, so I fell against the wrought iron. I fell diagonally, badly enough that I had an eight-inch laceration where the metal sliced deep into my back.

"By the time I went to bed that night, my neck was stiff. I had a very difficult time turning it to the right. By the time I woke up in the morning, I couldn't move my head at all, and my breathing was very shallow. My parents just assumed I had a cold, so my mom treated it with wintergreen and camphor, rubbing it into my neck and putting a cotton baby diaper over it."

These symptoms persisted, and after several days Angela's parents took her to their family physician, who specialized in conditions of the ear, nose, and throat. A beloved and respected friend of the family, he told them she had tight muscles, that they were treating it properly, and that it would fade with the passage of time. Given the nature of his training, that may have been a reasonable conclusion for the doctor to reach.

Unfortunately, it was dead wrong. While a chiropractor would immediately suspect a causal relationship between the injury and the symptoms that developed so soon thereafter, such an idea never occurred to the medical physician. Angela had to live with the consequences.

"I had never had a stiff neck before, but they all assumed I had caught a draft. They never connected it with the fall at school. From that point on, my breathing was always impaired. I had noticed, and told Mom and Dad, that I had a hard time breathing deeply and that it *hurt*, in the chest but mostly in the back. It was a pulling sensation and a restriction. None of these conditions had been present before the fall."

Further complications continued to develop:

"After the fall, I became very prone to kidney and bladder infections. I never had any infections before the fall. There was no propensity toward this, no family history of kidney and bladder disorders. The doctor said I'd outgrow it."

Once again, the doctor's rosy predictions were way off the mark. Through her teens and early twenties, Angela's urinary tract problems worsened considerably:

> "I'd start with low-grade fevers and nausea. There would be a burning sensation whenever I would urinate and an incredible itching through the whole urethra area. Just incredible, indescribable. The worst part, when it was severe, was pain like razor blades. All those symptoms would become very exaggerated, and I would sometimes vomit or just get the dry heaves. Later, as things worsened, I would go into spasms and convulsions and would pass out. Also, my skin was terribly discolored."

Angela had uremic poisoning, a condition in which the body is poisoned by its own waste matter. Having treated her urinary problems for several years with standard medications, Angela's family physician eventually realized the case was getting out of control. After an incident in which she passed out while driving a car, he referred her to one of the most highly regarded medical clinics in the Midwest.

The specialist who treated Angela there, a well-respected physician second-in-charge at the clinic, told her the disorder was incurable. They could maintain her on certain strong medications for a while longer, he said, but she would be on a dialysis machine within two years. With the certainty of an expert, he told her to prepare for this inevitable course of events. Angela was stunned, but unwilling to accept the doctor's verdict:

> "I was twenty-five, and I wanted to live a normal life. I was really determined not to let his prediction come true. I had to go into the clinic every week to get blood checks and urine checks. That I could deal with, but not the idea of having to get dialysis for the rest of my life. I mean, he clearly said I wouldn't lead a normal life. He told me I should plan on not having children, because my own life would be endangered."

At the darkest hour, help came from an unexpected source.

Angela's college roommate's mother had studied the Edgar Cayce readings for years and suggested an alternative:

> "She said, 'Sweetie, you need to get to a chiropractor. I'm going to get this Cayce information for you and I want you to read it. We cured our cat of an "incurable" kidney disorder, and she's living today. I want you to take this information, and I want you to pull out of it what you can, and apply it in your life.'
>
> "With the cat, my roommate's mother had used high quantities of vitamins A, E, and C and had also taken it to her chiropractor. She said to me, 'I know the same treatment will help you.' I read through the two volumes of Cayce material. I could barely understand Cayce, but I got through it. What I was able to understand was that I needed a chiropractor. I didn't know where to find one, but I decided to do it. The other part of it was to take the vitamins. Also, the Cayce information said I should drink no carbonated beverages or alcohol and eat no refined white products like sugar and white flour. In college, I had gotten into the habit of drinking ten or twelve sodas a day, so this was going to be a big change."

Back in the mid-1960s, these health recommendations seemed far more radical than they would today. The phrase "junk food" was not yet part of the American vocabulary, and the idea that nutrition could have a major effect on the healing of disease had virtually no support in the mainstream medical community. The holistic health revolution still lay in the future, and Angela was entering what was then relatively uncharted territory.

As things turned out, Angela didn't go to a chiropractor. No one she knew had been to one, and she was concerned about going to any doctor who hadn't been personally recommended. But she did drastically alter her diet, following the recommendations in the Cayce information she had read. After eating a diet high in sugar and fat for her entire life, Angela completely eliminated junk food, replacing it with whole grains, fruits, vegetables, fish, and poultry.

She remembers feeling a pronounced physical shift almost immediately, an inner knowing that her body was using the new foods to correct the severe imbalance it had confronted for so many years. It was as if her body were heaving a big sigh of relief at being provided the raw material it needed to function normally. Within a week, she felt so much better that she started to wean herself from the prescription medication. Angela did not mention this to anyone.

"I told no one, because I was weak enough that I knew I could be persuaded not to follow through. And something from inside was driving me, saying, 'Do it! Do it!' I didn't have any encouragement from anyone. I hadn't even called back the friends who had introduced me to the information. It was a solo thing for me."

While support from friends is one of the most important things in life, sometimes we feel compelled to act alone. In doing so, we learn a great deal about our own inner strength. The great turning points in our lives often spring from just such situations—the ones for which we would almost never volunteer, but which allow us to discover our ability to rise to the occasion.

Within six weeks of changing her diet, Angela was in total remission.

"I knew something was different at the clinic, because they kept me for two hours one week and three hours the next, running all sorts of extra tests on me. But nobody was telling me what was going on.

"I was feeling great! I knew I hadn't been running any fever. But I didn't know what the urinalysis and blood tests were showing."

Though at that point in her life Angela was not in the habit of asserting herself with authority figures, she finally confronted the doctor in charge, demanding to know what was going on.

"He sat at his desk, shaking his head back and forth in a negative gesture. He said, 'I don't understand this.'

"I said, 'What don't you understand?'

"The doctor replied, 'There's no logical reason why this condition has cleared up. You are in complete remission. You're not spilling any blood, and there's no pus in the urine. We don't understand this. That's why we ran the tests, and reran them and reran them.' He said, 'You are clean, you are clear, and we don't have any reason.'

"I said, 'I'm cured! I'm all right!' I was absolutely elated.

"He said, 'You're fine. We don't understand this.'

"I said, 'I understand it. I understand it!' I told him about the dietary changes and the fact that I had gone out on a limb and weaned myself from all the medication.

"The doctor kept saying, 'I don't understand.'

"I said, 'I understand! I have found another way to take control and to take charge of my life. I have a future now, without the dialysis machine, without medication, and without all that dependency.' "

Angela told him the whole story. Ludicrous as it all sounded to her at first, she had gone ahead with the dietary changes out of a desperate desire for her life to return to normal. She told the doctor, "I'm too young to live the kind of life that you described."

Then she asked her doctor what to her was a perfectly logical question: "Doesn't this warrant your doing some research?"

"Absolutely not," the doctor replied without skipping a beat. "My training does not allow for this kind of thinking or this form of regime. I could not recommend it to anybody, nor research it."

Angela was stunned and outraged.

"I was infuriated that I had healed myself after he had told me it was impossible, and now he wouldn't even use this information to help other people. Here's someone who has the authority, the power, and the position. He's running a multimillion dollar operation, one considered to be second only to the Mayo Clinic in that part of the country. I was infuriated and dumbfounded. I pursued it a second

time, and he gave me the same pat answer. And I said,
'That's a poor excuse, because it has worked for me.' His
answer was, 'You're only one person. There are many variables, and you are only one person.' "

Angela never convinced the doctor to change his mind. But
her own life was deeply changed by the experience. And there
was more to come.

Ten years later, she was a schoolteacher, living in Virginia
Beach, Virginia. On summer vacation, she traveled to the American Northwest with her mother, Jeanette, and a friend, Sonia.
    They had just stopped for gas in Spokane, Washington, and
were on their way to Glacier National Park. Sonia was driving,
Jeanette was in the front passenger seat, and Angela had just gone
to sleep in the back seat. She wanted to be well rested when her
turn came to drive a few hours later.
    Both Angela and her mother had concerns about the trip, mis-
givings they had shared with each other. Believers in the power
of intuition, they had jointly decided earlier that day to discon-
tinue the trip and head back home. But Sonia wanted to keep
going. Angela and Jeanette, with nothing other than their intuition on which to base their change of heart, relented.
    It was a fateful decision. Disobeying a strong message from
one's inner voice is rarely advisable, but disappointing a friend
was more than Angela and her mother felt able to do that day.

    "On the day we left Spokane, as we were leaving the gas
station, I had one foot in the car, getting into the back seat,
and something said, 'Get up and drive! Don't go to sleep!' It
was loud and shocking, like a dagger going through my
whole body. I put my foot back out of the car and said,
'Sonia, I'm going to drive.'
    "She said, 'No, no, no. You're tired; you need to rest.' I
said, 'Sonia, I'm going to drive.' And the voice again inside
me said, 'DRIVE! Don't let her drive; you drive. Don't go to
sleep.'
    "Sonia said, 'No, Angela, come on. I'll just drive a little

while longer. You need to get a little more sleep, because you're not real fresh to take the wheel.' She made perfect sense, because I was tired. She said, 'I know this area real well, and you don't.' And I said, 'O.K., all right, I'll take over in a couple of hours.' I got in the back seat, and that's the last I remember."

Shortly thereafter, their vehicle spun out of control on the foggy mountain road, crashing into a tree. The next thing Angela recalls is seeing her own body on the ground, from a vantage point somewhere above it:

"The next thing I knew, I was hovering over my body. I was terribly confused, seeing my body on the ground at that point. I heard somebody say, 'We've got to get help,' and another person said they had already radioed for help. I can remember my mother saying repeatedly, 'Don't die. Don't die, Angela, don't die.' Every time she would say it, it was like a physical sword piercing my body.

"At the same time I was feeling, 'This is wonderful! I don't need all that.' I knew that my physical body had gone through a lot of trauma, though at that point I didn't know exactly what kind, because I wasn't focusing on that. I just was astonished at this separation and this freedom that I was experiencing. I said, 'I'm going on. I really don't want this any more.' I kept hearing my mother imploring me not to die, but I said to myself, 'I've got to go on.'

"I looked down at those people and saw what they were doing to my body. One woman started giving mouth-to-mouth resuscitation, and another started pushing on my chest and it hurt. I said to myself, 'I don't need to let this hurt any more. I'm just going on.' I heard them say, 'I think she's gone. She's not responding.' I could hear sirens in the distance, and all around me I saw darkness.

"It was very dark, but I was moving. I could feel my whole essence moving forward. I saw a pinpoint of light ahead of me, and I said, 'This is what I have always heard about. This is fantastic. There's no pain. I'm free. I'm totally free. The closer I got to the light, the more it imbued me.

"I stopped a couple of times, because I kept responding to my mother's call, which was like a magnet. I didn't want it; I wanted to repel it. I looked back and saw my body being put on a stretcher and carried to an ambulance. My mother was next to me, trying to reach out to me and hold my hand.

"I remember hearing this siren, and I looked at my body and I knew there was some life there . . . I merged with the body momentarily and I thought, 'This is more pain than this body can handle.' The sound of the siren and the movement of the vehicle made my head feel as if it were being slit into many pieces. My ears and my skull were unbelievably painful.

"So I said, 'Over and out. This is not for me.' I moved toward the light, and I was almost totally one with this light when a voice said, 'No! You have to stop. You can't go on.' I said, 'No, I'm not!' It said, 'You must stop. It's not your time. You must go back.' I said, 'Please, this is what I always thought it was like. This is more wonderful than I read about and thought about. I'm ready to go on. I really want to work on the other side.' The voice said, 'It's not your time. You have more that is yet to be done on the earth plane.' I said, 'Please!' but the voice was insistent, 'You must go back.' "

This realm beyond the physical, so vividly experienced by Angela, has been extensively chronicled by Raymond Moody, M.D., Ph.D., in his ground-breaking book, *Life After Life*.[1] Angela's near-death experience (NDE) shows marked similarities to those of thousands of other people from all walks of life.

Dr. Moody, a psychiatrist and college professor, has devoted much of his professional life to exploring the NDE. When I interviewed Moody, I asked him how, as a scientifically trained physician, he came to accept the NDE as something more than oxygen deprivation to the brain. He replied that he had reached the conclusion gradually, as he examined more and more cases which forced him to re-evaluate his preconceptions:

"When I first heard about this, I assumed it was something like a shock to the brain and so forth. I know many physicians, literally from all over the world, who have investigated this phenomenon, and they all started with that assumption. All of us, in talking with the people who have had these experiences, have come around very much in our views.

"The classic definition of an hallucination, of course, is that it's an apparent sensory experience without a corresponding external event. That is, a person sees or hears something when there is not really anything there. But with these near-death experiences, we have many cases where the patients, while they are out of their bodies, are able to witness something going on at a distance, even in another part of the hospital, which later turns out by independent verification to have been exactly as the patient said. So this is very difficult to put together with a simple physiological or biochemical explanation.

"Another thing that makes me feel that the experience is something beyond just an hallucination is the profound effects these experiences have on people. They have this complete confidence that what we call death is just a passage into another level of reality.

"I think that no final answer, though, can be settled on because ultimately in this frontier area of the human mind, there aren't any experts that can give us the answer. There is no conventionally established way yet to determine the answer. Everybody is going to have to look at this and make up his own mind in his own way. All I can do is speak for myself and my many colleagues in medicine who have looked into this, and we're all convinced that the patients do get a glimpse of the beyond."[2]

Angela's breath-taking glimpse of the beyond was immediately followed by a crashing, painful return to physical reality:

"Going back into my body felt awful, beyond any pain that I had ever experienced. It was awful, because it was something more than physical. I just didn't want to come back. I really didn't. It was very hard to merge back into my body, so I didn't. I stayed out of it, just hovering above it. My breath was very shallow.

"I was able to scan my body like an x-ray machine. My brain tissue appeared swollen, and I went through the rest of the body and saw that I had sustained most of the injuries on the right side. The right hip, rib cage, ovary, and shoulder. There were no lacerations as such, except on the scalp. I just kept looking and saying to myself how interesting it all was.

"My right shoulder and hip sustained the most pressure, as did my head. At any rate, what I remember next is being in a hallway in a hospital. I would regain consciousness and then lose it again. I was hovering all the time, because I couldn't handle what the physical body was going through. I just wanted to do what I had to for this physical body and then go back out again. I also knew something had happened to my overall ability to communicate, because I could hardly speak at all. I didn't know what had happened, but I perceived that it had something to do with my endocrine system."

Aside from the injuries just mentioned, Angela was informed by her doctor that she also had a concussion with brain contusions. In addition, her inner ears had been shaken by the force of hitting her head on the side of the car, so she felt as though she were in an echo chamber.

"I was constantly dizzy and had double vision. My balance was totally off, whether I was sitting, standing, or lying down. All movement was upsetting to my system. I was very traumatized, so much so that if I heard a horn blow outside, I would start shuddering and shaking. I couldn't control that. I couldn't hold down solid foods, due to nausea. I had little to no use of my right leg and arm. I just couldn't move them, from the bruising. I could not lift my arm forward or sideways. It just hung there. And my right leg was mostly numb."

After a couple of weeks, she was sent back to her parents' home in the Midwest, where she stayed for four months, using crutches the whole time. She also experienced partial amnesia, in which significant portions of her memory remained inaccessible.

Shortly after arriving at her parents', she had her first menstrual period since the accident.

> "I passed out from the pain. It wasn't just cramping. There was a pain that came from the right rib cage all around my back, and I couldn't even breathe. My sister and my dad found me passed out in the bathroom. The pains were just intolerable. They immediately called the family physician, and then he called in a gynecologist."

The family physician had no definite explanation and expressed concern that Angela might be having a gall bladder attack. The gynecologist felt the pain was related to her ovary, which had been bruised in the automobile accident. When her period ended, the worst of the pain subsided, but she lived in dread of her next menses. This was just part of her problem, however. The aftereffects of the accident were severe, and it was several weeks before Angela could walk, even with assistance.

> "Day after day for many weeks, my sister and my father had to help me get to the bathroom. I just couldn't walk, because of the dizziness and the immobility. It was two years before I could walk normally again. I was on crutches, and then used a cane for over a year and a half. I was so traumatized that I wouldn't get into a car for almost two years, unless family or friends were driving me to the chiropractor or to the physical therapist."

Regular chiropractic adjustments were part of Angela's rehabilitation program, and she feels this played a crucial role in enabling her to walk again. Angela also saw a psychiatrist for her amnesia, which was diagnosed as selective amnesia. Her dizziness and double vision lasted over a year and a half, and her memory returned fully in two years. It took longer for the shoulder and hip pain to ease, but eventually these, too, were gone.

The one symptom that persisted, nightmarish in its intensity, was the excruciating pain just below the right rib cage for the several days around her period each month.

"For that whole time, whenever I would have a period, it was like a crucifixion. The intense rib cage pain—I couldn't control it at all. At the point when I returned to Virginia Beach, there were two or three specialists called in. Each had a different diagnosis, and none had a lasting solution."

Highly motivated to find a solution, Angela tried every available method, orthodox and unorthodox, in pursuit of healing. None of them offered more than temporary, partial relief. To function during this monthly torture, Angela experimented with her diet. Eventually she discovered by trial and error that if she ate nothing but fruits and vegetables for the few days preceding her period, the pain would not be quite as severe.

She had read that eating lighter foods like fruits and vegetables places less stress on the digestive system than heavy fare like meats and fried foods. Fruits and vegetables are digested quickly, thus minimizing the level of metabolic activity in the abdominal area, where her pain was so pronounced. But even this provided only minimal relief, so she took six to eight ibuprofen (Advil®) tablets a day before her period and twelve to twenty a day during the peak days.

Taking medication like this ran contrary to her natural healing philosophy, but under the circumstances she felt she had no choice. Even these large doses of medication sometimes weren't enough to mask the pain.

When Angela eventually found her way to my office, fourteen years after the motor vehicle accident that had altered her life so dramatically, she never even mentioned the trouble with her menstrual period. She had other things on her mind. A few months earlier, she had slipped while scrubbing a bathtub, twisting her back while reaching in vain for a towel rack in an attempt to keep from falling. She was almost completely bedridden at home for weeks. But since she was uninsured and in financial difficulty, she had not sought professional help.

"I couldn't stand, I couldn't sit, I was in pain, and my lower back was spasming constantly. I had completely lost feeling in my right hand. Those things had been with me on and off through the years since the automobile accident. But now this incredible pain and the immobility from it were overwhelming, and I started to lose feeling in both big toes. Within a month after the fall, I noticed that the front of my left thigh was feeling as if it wasn't getting full circulation. It felt cool all the time, with pins and needles."

The day before she called me, Angela felt a shot of intense pain in her lower back and fell to the floor. As she slowly arose, she realized she could no longer delay seeking help. Since she had severe financial problems, I offered to treat her free of charge, and she agreed. When she filled in the new patient information form at her first visit to my office, Angela said she wanted treatment for "lower back pain; right foot pain; numbness in both hands and left thigh."

As I examined Angela, it seemed to me that from a chiropractic standpoint, so many things were abnormal that it wasn't easy to know where to begin. The numbness in both arms and legs, combined with other physical findings, led me to proceed with great caution, since there was a possibility that one or more spinal discs were herniated. In particular, I found that when a pinwheel was passed across the top of her right foot, she could barely feel it. This is generally a sign of nerve pressure or irritation in the lower back, because the nerves from the lower spine are the source of all nerve supply to the legs. Getting an MRI scan to rule out a disc involvement would have been helpful, but that was an impossibility because of the cost involved.

Noting these limitations, I began with very light adjustments to her neck and lower back, hoping these would begin the recovery process. With Angela lying on her back, I used my hands to gently apply a tractioning force on her neck and found that doing so relieved some of the pain in both her neck and lower back. I used the pelvic blocking technique I described in earlier chapters and also adjusted the uppermost joint in her neck on the specialized side posture table. I decided to wait before attempting any other manipulations, so that I could monitor the response to these initial therapies.

When Angela returned for her second visit two days later, she was still in pain, but said that she had been able to sleep through the night without interruption for the first time since the bathtub accident four months earlier. She also described a new-found feeling of ease and peace.

Seeing a positive response to my initial approach, I used additional manipulative methods at the second visit, including the flexion-distraction technique. This method, originally developed by Raymond McManis, D.O., an early twentieth-century osteopath, and brought to the attention of modern chiropractors by James Cox, D.C., utilizes an adjusting table with which the doctor can apply traction in three planes of motion. It is used to treat disorders of the lower back, including spinal disc protrusions. At her next visit, Angela reported a decrease in lower back pain and arm numbness. Over the next few weeks, I added further treatments, including adjustments of the second and third cervical vertebrae. Improvement continued.

She recalls it this way:

"I regained feeling in my toes and in the left thigh. Lifting my legs was still difficult, but rapidly my whole body felt as if it had more agility. I could raise my arms without pain. My neck had far more mobility and no spasms. I was able to drive my car without having the numbness penetrate throughout the lower part of my arms. The real revelation to me was the progress with my lower back. I could bend and I could pick things up. I couldn't believe it—the healing was on all levels."

Aside from the decreased levels of pain, Angela also described feeling "reconnected to my body." For the first time in many years, she was able to sit peacefully in meditation. On some occasions, she had a sense of energy moving up and down her spine, something she had experienced in the past, but not since the automobile accident fourteen years earlier.

I have had other patients with back or neck injuries who have reported improvement in their ability to meditate as a result of chiropractic treatment. While the exact mechanism by which this occurs is a matter of speculation, it is worth noting that meditation teachers emphasize the importance of assuming a straight-backed posture during meditation. Generally this means either sitting up straight or lying flat on one's back, although other positions such as walking or running also meet this criterion.

As our knowledge of the meditative process (see Chapter Thirteen) is enhanced through research in the coming years, we may come to better understand the spine's role in the process, in terms of nerve transmission and energetic flows. Until then, we can ponder the anecdotal evidence from people like Angela, whose experiential reports provide clues of a relationship between spinal balance and enhancement of the meditative process.

At Angela's third visit, I checked the polarity reflex points on her toes. Certain points on the feet are believed to relate to other organs and systems, and a toe that is particularly painful to pressure may indicate a problem elsewhere in the body. The polarity system from India, like that of traditional Chinese medicine, speaks of "elements," with names like earth, water, and fire. These elements have both physical and emotional correlates, and indicate patterns of balance or imbalance within the body-mind complex.

In Angela's case, when I pressed on her toes, they all felt pretty much the same to her, except for the third toe on the right side. Pressure on that one nearly sent her to the ceiling.

"What was that?" she asked, startled.

"I need to take a look at something else," I replied, "and then I'll be glad to talk about it." Knowing that the polarity system considers the third toe a diagnostic reflex point for the fire element and that the fire element relates to an energetic center in the area of the solar plexus (mid-abdomen), I went directly to the area on the right side of the abdomen just below the rib cage and pressed there.

Angela jumped. "How did you know?" she wondered aloud, adding, "I should have told you before. That's the area where I have this horrible pain every time I menstruate. It's been that way since the accident."

That's how I found out about her menstrual pain. She had been so preoccupied dealing with the aftereffects of the fall in the tub that she had neglected to mention this other problem.

In polarity therapy, there are specific contacts recommended for dealing with imbalances in each of the elements. For the fire element, these contacts are at the top of the head, the solar plexus or mid-back, and the thigh. These contacts are treated with a gentle rocking motion, and I treated Angela in these areas. As conceived in the Indian healing methods, the fire element has many manifestations, among them the sense of personal power and self-assertion, the function of the digestive system, and the craving or dislike for hot, spicy foods.

I asked Angela if she craved hot, spicy foods.

"As a matter of fact, I love them. I can sometimes eat jalapeño peppers by the jarful if I let myself."

"Have you had any recently?" I queried.

"No, I haven't. I'd love to, but I'm not sure they're good for me. I've read some books on nutrition that aren't too enthusiastic about them." This was a well-read, knowledgeable, health-care consumer I was speaking with. But books don't always tell the whole story.

"Books can only speak in general terms," I told her. "Each person is an individual. If you like jalapeño peppers, I want you to feel free to indulge yourself for a while. Have as many as you want. And if you want to have Mexican or other ethnic foods that fill the craving, go for it! I have a feeling it's going to be very good for you. It looks as if we need to 'feed your fire.'"

I know people who, if they eat one bite of a hot pepper, will have severe digestive upset for weeks. But others thrive on them. To generalize about which foods are good and which are bad can be valuable, but only insofar as we bear in mind that these are just generalizations. All rules have their exceptions, and some people's bodies seem to play by different rules than others.

Angela had her next menstrual period twelve days later. It was her least painful period in the fourteen years since the automobile accident and the first one in five years when she hadn't needed any ibuprofen for the pain. For her to go from a dozen or more pills a day to zero was far beyond my expectations. She, too, was astonished and thrilled. By the time another month had passed, Angela had experienced the first pain-free menses of her entire life. To say she was pleased would be the understatement of the year. As of a year and a half later, her periods had remained pain-free and normal.

Since my work with Angela was not a controlled study, I don't have any way of knowing how much of the improvement in her dysmenorrhea is attributable to the dietary changes and how much to the chiropractic and polarity work. I do know from other cases in my own practice and from the reports of many other chiropractors that there are numerous instances where chiropractic adjustments alone can bring about a substantial improvement in cases of dysmenorrhea. Generally, this is in response to adjustment of the lower back, from which nerves branch out to supply the uterus and other internal organs of the pelvis.

There have been two controlled clinical studies in which spinal manipulation effects on dysmenorrhea were studied. In each, the response was quite promising.[3,4] There is also substantial documentation from holistic medical physicians and others, testifying to the positive effects of various dietary changes in cases of dysmenorrhea. Magnesium and vitamin B_6 are prominent among the nutrients with scientifically demonstrated positive effects for both dysmenorrhea and premenstrual syndrome.[5]

Angela's other symptoms cleared gradually over a period of four months, during which time I treated her on an intensive basis, seeing her two or three times a week. Her lower back pain and hand numbness receded to the point where they were no longer major factors in her life. Sometimes under the physical stress of her work cleaning houses, Angela's lower back would again become painful or the numbness would intensify in her right hand. But these symptoms did not again become so severe that she had to build her life around them for extended periods of time.

After two years, she still receives chiropractic treatment once

or twice a month, and is gradually decreasing her frequency of
visits.

* * *

Angela's dramatic tale raises many questions and provides
some answers as well. One of the most frustrating parts of being
a chiropractor is seeing people who were treated with standard
medical techniques, going downhill for years, enduring significant pain and hardship, when chiropractic or nutritional
methods could have spared their travail.

If Angela hadn't found out that an alternative approach existed, she would have been dependent on a kidney dialysis
machine from age twenty-five onward. She was fortunate. How
many others have not been so fortunate? The almost unbeliev-
able arrogance of the physician who refused to even explore this
alternative is deeply disturbing and is not unique. Angela was not
asking the physician to forsake his medical practice, become a
devotee of a psychic diagnostician, and thereby possibly risk losing all he had worked so hard to achieve. All she was asking was
that, as a professional whose goal was the good health of his patients, he should explore the factors which had apparently
brought about a complete cure in a case he had confidently
deemed incurable.

Perhaps, as the doctor apparently assumed, such research
would demonstrate that eliminating cola drinks, eating whole
foods, and taking certain vitamins would have no consistent effect on cases similar to Angela's. On the other hand, perhaps it
would have shown that half the sample group showed no improvement, forty-five percent benefited moderately, and five
percent were completely cured. Such research findings would
not justify touting these therapeutic measures as a sure-fire cure,
but wouldn't they be worth knowing about? Suppose you were
one of the five percent or fifty percent who would avert dependence on a dialysis machine through these simple, inexpensive
methods. Wouldn't this be something you'd like to be told?

The doctor's attitude was more than close-minded; it was also

profoundly unscientific. Science, properly practiced, is fundamentally just and democratic, neither endorsing nor rejecting
out of hand any new hypothesis. Instead, the scientific mind
seeks to concoct a test which will prove a hypothesis true or false.
In the democracy of science, all hypotheses are innocent until
proven guilty.

It is true that some hypotheses lend themselves to quantita-
tive measurement more easily than others. But it seems to me
that a study in which uremic patients were forbidden to drink
soda pop and eat sugar-laden products would have been fairly
straightforward, not difficult at all to construct. Equally significant, it would not have endangered people in either the control
group or the test group. But it could only have been run by a physician who had access to those patients.

Unfortunately, a tunnel-vision focus on the use of medications
to decrease or eliminate symptoms can point a doctor in precisely the wrong direction. There is an old cliché which says that
if your only tool is a hammer, you will see nails everywhere. Similarly, if your entire therapeutic approach is geared to the
pharmaceutical treatment of disease, you will tend to reject alternative approaches and may therefore overlook some causative
factors that underlie the disease.

It is appalling that a specialist in diseases of the urinary system could carry on blissfully unaware that drinking a dozen colas
a day might impact negatively on the urinary tract. Common
sense, if not atrophied by education and specialization, leads one
to look at the substances that are passing through an area that is
becoming irritated. When the process is external, as with inflam-
mations of the skin, anyone with a whit of sense knows enough
to think back on whether he or she might have rubbed up against
some poison oak or used some new hand cream or household
chemical. But when the process is going on inside the body, this
logic often vanishes.

I wish I could say that the passage of time since Angela had
her urinary disease has rendered such myopic thinking a thing of
the past. Sadly, I can't. I am generally a hopeful, optimistic person, and I do note changes for the better, but not nearly enough.
Patients like Dolores and Jimmy, whom you read about earlier in

this book, faced similar problems with their physicians in just the past few years. Their diseases differed from Angela's, but the "medicate-the-symptom" approach with which they were treated was exactly the same. The underlying causes of their ailments were ignored, and the results were no better.

Angela's story also contains a message about the role of intuition in the healing arts. My own diagnostic approach to this case differed in certain respects from the way I approach most other patients. In particular, my decision to test the polarity reflex points, which led me to unearth her right-sided abdominal sensitivity and menstrual pain, was largely intuitive. I don't use this test with all patients, and I frankly can't offer a specific set of diagnostic factors that led me to use it with Angela. It just felt intuitively right.

When I interviewed Dr. Norman Shealy, the founder and former president of the American Holistic Medical Association, I asked him about the role of intuition in diagnosis. He said, "Probably every time you see a patient, it's your intuition that tells you what tests to do. It really isn't just facts. You can choose among ten thousand different options." Finally, when all is said and done, the role of the doctor is to master a discipline as fully as possible and then allow intuition to work through the channel of that discipline.

The healing arts are arts, not just sciences. The more a doctor recognizes the importance of the intuitive aspects of diagnosis, the more likely he or she will be to listen closely. And as one listens more closely, the likelihood increases that what is said will be heard clearly. Nothing decreases the chance of spotting unexpected diagnostic information more than a mind that is already made up. Being a good listener is more than just common courtesy; it is the best single way to access the whole picture, or at least a large enough part of it to point your treatments in the right direction.

Poets have long known that, as songwriter John Stewart puts it, "they are only radio receivers, and the songs are really coming from somewhere else." In the creative arts, it has always been fully acceptable to call on the muse for inspiration and to freely admit to the power of one's intuitive side. In our society, it is far less acceptable for doctors to admit this, because it seems to imply an admission that science does not have all the answers. This, in turn, tarnishes the aura of certainty so carefully cultivated by the medical professions.

Let me be as clear about this as I possibly can. I am fully in favor of professionals staying up-to-date on scientific developments. But I also feel we would do ourselves, and society at large, a great favor by coming clean about the vast uncertainties within which all healing arts operate. We are never going to fully understand the workings of the human body, just as we are never going to fully understand the creation of the universe. There is a grand mystery of which we are but a small part, and retaining a measure of awe in the face of it all is a stance to be honored, not discouraged.

There remains one part of Angela's recovery I haven't yet touched upon. Several weeks into the changes she experienced while under my care, she told me that she felt "on purpose" for the first time in many years. She took out an unfinished book manuscript on child development and over several months completed it.

I find it difficult to credit this turnaround to my treatment. But to Angela, there was no question about it. The energetic shift she experienced as a result of her physical healing led to a sense of inner renewal, culminating in her feeling reinspired to complete a demanding task requiring sharp mental focus and a keen sense of purpose.

When we closely examine the hazy interfaces of body, mind, and spirit, the notion of direct cause and effect no longer stands out in sharp relief. Certain aspects of the healing process, particularly when that process goes deep, remain wholly outside the realm of the measurable. Yet these may be the most significant markers of true healing. It is one of the grand paradoxes of our time that as medical science's capacity for micromeasurement has multiplied manifold, so, too, has our awareness that areas forever outside its domain are crucial to health and healing.

CHAPTER 6

DAVID'S BRIDGE

David came to me for help with his neck, shoulder, and upper back pain. An automobile accident three years earlier had left him with low-grade nagging pain in those areas, an ongoing reminder of the whiplash he had sustained.

A university student whose academic pursuits included religion, philosophy, and psychology, David had heard me sing at a massage therapy school graduation ceremony several weeks before making an appointment to see me. On the line where my intake form asks, "Referred by?" he wrote "No one; hey, enjoyed your tunes!" I liked him immediately, not only because he enjoyed my music, but because something about him reminded me of myself a couple of decades earlier.

The physical aspects of his case history were typical of a whiplash injury for which chiropractic care was needed but had never been provided. The area between his upper neck and mid-back was always at least mildly uncomfortable, and when he stayed in one position too long or engaged in stressful physical activity, it worsened. Also noteworthy was the fact that he smoked more than a pack of cigarettes each day. Nicotine, which causes blood vessels to constrict, can contribute to chronic muscle tension by depriving the muscles of their normal blood supply.

David had a part-time job which required a great deal of talking on the telephone, and at the end of a workday he felt quite sore, not only in the neck, shoulder, and upper back, but also in the muscles on the left side of his lower back.

He also volunteered that he was in the middle of an emotionally stressful time due to the recent breakup of a love relationship. As the relationship with his girlfriend was falling apart, he experienced a marked increase in neck and back pain, along with the appearance of new areas of discomfort in his abdomen and chest. He told me that when the emotional tension was most pronounced, he found it difficult to breathe deeply, and I noticed that his breathing was mildly labored as we spoke. The physical pain, combined with the emotional unease, had also made it difficult for him to sleep at night for the preceding few weeks.

I appreciated David's openness about these personal matters and made a mental note to follow up on them. I then proceeded to do my standard first-visit physical, looking for clues that might enable me to help fix the aches and pains that had brought him to me.

When I examined David's spine, there was evidence of mild to moderate chronic muscle strain in the neck and upper back, with spinal subluxations in both areas. His muscles were well-developed and well-toned, but there was a greater than normal degree of tension along the right side of his neck, in the trapezius muscle (part of which runs between the neck and the shoulder), and in the muscles surrounding his right shoulder blade. The second and third cervical vertebrae in his neck were markedly restricted in mobility, as were the fourth and fifth thoracic vertebrae between the shoulder blades.

Fortunately, the examination revealed no signs of nerve damage, and since his overall posture and muscle tone were better than average, I hoped for and expected a satisfactory response to treatment. I suggested that we see each other twice the first week and base the treatment frequency after that on the response to those initial sessions. I expected that he would be much improved within a couple of weeks, but adopted a wait-and-see attitude because I wanted to be sure not to overpromise.

The first adjustment I gave David was a rotational manipulation of the joint where the second and third cervical vertebrae meet, with him in a seated position. I explained before I adjusted him, as I always do before using this particular maneuver for the first time with a patient, that it probably would not hurt, but that the feeling might be surprising.

I showed him the position I would use, with my hands gently holding his head, and explained that the rotational movement would cover a very small arc, "not a 360- or a 180-, more like a 5- to 10-degree arc." I find that many people who have watched the movie, *The Exorcist*, in which a young girl's head spins all the way around, have internalized a fear that chiropractic adjustments will bear some unwelcome similarity. This is, of course, untrue. Mentioning that it's "not a 360-degree or a 180-degree" usually breaks the ice, provoking a smile or laughter, thus allowing increased relaxation when it's most needed.

When I adjusted David's second and third cervical vertebrae, a loud pop could be heard across the room. He said, "Wow!" and sat quietly for a few moments. Then he reported that the tension in his neck was almost entirely gone. I asked if I had accurately described how the adjustment would feel, and he confirmed that it had indeed been surprising, but also completely painless.

Then I had him lie face down on one of my chiropractic tables and adjusted the fourth and fifth vertebrae in his upper back, massaging the muscles in that area immediately afterward to preempt the possibility of a reflexive muscle spasm. Then, as he lay on his back, I applied a basic polarity therapy contact to aid the relaxation of his neck muscles. I cradled the back of his head in my hands, pressing the middle finger of each hand into the soft valley where the top of the neck meets the occiput bone in the back of the skull. Generally, I hold this contact until I feel a strong sensation of heat in my contact fingers.

Within a few seconds of my making the contact, David started to shake all over. I thought he was cold and brought over a blanket to cover him. I asked if he were all right, and he said, "Yes, I am." Then I resumed the contact. Here's how he described the experience four months later:

> "I was shaking like crazy, but I wasn't cold. It was as if something that I had been stomping down in myself, intentionally or otherwise, had been released or unblocked. All of a sudden, it was as if all these energies, which would normally get stuck in my neck, were moving through my whole body. I specifically remember what felt like a current of energy just racing up and down my neck. I also remember seeing beautiful colors, lots of blues and greens. It was like a trail of lights. I can just picture them, going up and down my back in a clockwise motion. I had not previously experienced anything like that, ever."

David's journey had only begun. The almost psychedelic beauty and the rush of energy soon gave way to a darker vision:

> "It was as if I had been torn in two—this is purely mental—between the love for a woman and the need to be myself, without being controlled or manipulated. There was this chasm and just darkness in between."

The "purely mental" construct in the mind of this philosophy student quickly took on physical form.

> "There was the right side and the left side, and a black space between. I remember lying on the table, feeling my hands and my feet for what felt like the first time in my life. I don't remember exactly what the thoughts were, but it was a synthesis that said, 'Hey, both these sides are compatible, and here is the key to putting them together. Here is the little bridge.' And it just went *kwoossh*! And then there was no dichotomy between the right and the left. Whatever that chasm was, I bridged it. It just came together. I don't know exactly what that means in body-mind terminology, but I know it felt super, and it still does. It felt so incredibly good!"

Interestingly, the contact I applied at the back of David's upper neck is one which is said to foster the free flow of energy between the left and right sides of the body. Rarely have I seen such powerful confirmation of this effect.

The visual and experiential sense of bridging this gap then led David toward resolution of another gap in his life:

"Having that thought led me directly to another one. I had been through a divorce. My son was with me, and my ex-wife had been with a number of different men. I guess there was a part of me that was afraid of losing my son. And then I realized in a flash, 'I'm never going to lose him.' That thought was so absolute and so pure that it left no doubt whatsoever."

While David was going through this experience, I remained crouched at the head of the chiropractic table, holding the contact points on his upper neck. I had no clue as to the content of his experience, but it was clear from the shaking throughout his body that something powerful was at work. I stayed silent for the most part, not wanting to interfere with his process, but a couple of times I said something like, "That's fine—go with it if you want to," or, on seeing a tear in his eye, "It's O.K., let it out." I wanted him to feel safe and supported and free to pursue his path unimpeded. I was also hopeful that the combined physical and emotional release would help the physical ailments (muscular pain, breathing difficulties) that had led him to seek my help.

After twenty minutes or so, the shaking slowed to a mild quiver and his breathing grew slower and consistently deeper. I applied other contacts to calm and ground him. One of these involved placing my right hand over the sacrum bone at the bottom of his spine, while my left hand covered the crown of his head.

Following such an intense experience, I wanted to be certain that he was sufficiently grounded and stabilized to be able to drive home safely. I recommended that he take some time to relax and assimilate the experience, and I advised against any major activity that was not absolutely required. In the early days of chiropractic, patients were often advised to rest after their adjustments, and some practitioners still consider this advisable. In our modern, fast-paced world, it is not always very practical, and I generally save such advice for special situations like David's.

In the consultation room with me afterward, David was ecstatic, waxing eloquent about the need to liberate the mind through the direct experience of the body and about the wonderment of bridging the chasms that hold us back from the mystical experience of oneness. He was ready to climb every mountain and ford every stream. I have learned that these magic moments of high attunement do not last forever, so I decided to push into an area which, while certainly more mundane, was particularly important for David's healing process. I spoke to him about cigarettes.

As is true with all smokers I've met, there was in David's case a strong tie-in between smoking and emotional tension. Now that he was in the midst of what appeared to be a deep emotional breakthrough, I asked him to look closely at his actions. I did not demand that he cut back on smoking. Instead, I requested that whenever he took out a cigarette, he ask himself what feeling had immediately preceded his doing so. Was it fear? Anger? Joy? Desire? Failure?

I asked him to keep track of these feelings, to see if a pattern emerged. I believed that if he looked closely at the process leading up to his lighting up, he'd probably "just say no" more of the time.

Because cigarettes are legally marketed, we sometimes forget how destructive and insidious they are. It is well known that they contribute strongly to lung cancer and heart disease. It is less well known that they account for far more deaths in the U.S. each year than AIDS, alcohol, automobile accidents, homicide, suicide, heroin, crack cocaine, and all other illegal drugs combined. It is almost completely unknown to the general public that, in the words of Andrew Weil, M.D., a knowledgeable writer on the subject of drug use, "tobacco in the form of cigarettes is the most addictive drug in the world, even more addictive than heroin."[1]

In his book, *Natural Health, Natural Medicine,* Dr. Weil, a holistic physician who is a faculty member in the Division of Social Perspectives in Medicine at the University of Arizona College of Medicine, explains that "two factors account for this: the pharmacological power of nicotine, one of the strongest stimulants known, and the efficiency of smoking as a drug delivery system. Smoking puts drugs into the brain more directly than intravenous injection. Almost everyone who uses cigarettes is addicted, and the addiction is very difficult to break . . . It is also far and away the most serious form of drug abuse in our society, alongside which the abuse of illegal drugs pales into insignificance."[2]

I certainly hoped that David would give up smoking, or at least significantly cut down on the amount he smoked. Otherwise, in twenty or thirty years or less, he'd be a prime candidate for cancer or heart disease. But I trusted that if he were to continue on the path of physical and emotional healing upon which he had embarked, he would give up smoking in his own good time. For the moment, I chose to use his addiction as a productive tool for encouraging greater self-awareness.

In addition, I showed him an exercise to improve his breathing and help him relax. I suggested that he use it several times a day. An excellent way to start the morning, it can be used at any hour. Aside from filling the lungs with air, this exercise provides some good stretching for the back and legs as well. (See Figure 1, page 174).

When David returned for his second visit two days later, he noted improvement in many areas. He was now able to sleep with his head turned to the right, a position which had previously been too painful. His lower back felt normal for the first time in months, and he said that he felt more "centered" than he had in a long time. In addition, he expressed relief that he was able to breathe without any sense of cramping or restriction in his chest.

Chiropractic adjustments can affect the breathing process via three main pathways in the nervous system. First, the lungs and the tubes leading to them (the bronchi and bronchioles) derive their sympathetic nerve supply from the second through fifth thoracic nerves in the upper back. Since the sympathetics control the nerve supply to blood vessels, an adjustment of the fourth and fifth thoracic vertebrae may have a normalizing effect on the blood supply to the lungs.

The second nerve pathway affecting the breathing apparatus involves the vagus nerve, the tenth cranial nerve. In older anatomy texts, the vagus is referred to as the pneumogastric nerve, because it provides the parasympathetic nerve supply to a number of internal organs, including the lungs (pneumo) and the stomach (gastric). Chiropractors seem most often to influence the vagus as it passes through the upper neck, close to the first cervical vertebra, also known as the atlas vertebra.

The sympathetic and parasympathetic systems work in tandem. It's as if one pushes when the other pulls, with each system sharing responsibility for maintaining a state of homeostasis or balance. Parasympathetic stimulation causes contraction of the breathing passages, while sympathetic activity opens them. Free breathing depends on a proper balance between the two.

The third way spinal adjustments affect the breathing mechanism is via the phrenic nerve, which originates at the third, fourth, and fifth cervical vertebrae. This nerve travels from its site of origin in the neck, through the chest to the diaphragm, the large muscle that separates the chest from the abdomen. The phrenic nerve controls the muscular activity of the diaphragm, which is crucial to proper breathing. In David's first two visits, I adjusted all of the vertebral areas related to the lungs. After that, he experienced no further breathing difficulty.

During his second and third visits, I again applied the polarity contacts which had elicited so dramatic a response the first time, yet no shaking occurred at all. The blockage was nowhere to be found. Seeing this, I focused on chiropractic adjustments in areas of vertebral restriction, varying the angle of adjustment somewhat to be certain that freedom of joint motion in all directions was being restored. In addition, I used ultrasound and hot packs at the third visit to allow more complete release of the residual tension in David's neck muscles.

David's neck, shoulder, and back pain decreased quickly. Within three weeks, he was pain-free most of the time. I saw him six times the first month, adjusting the cervical and thoracic vertebrae when necessary and continuing polarity treatments.

During these treatments, David occasionally experienced powerful surges of energy and more frequently achieved a state of deep relaxation.

Between three and four weeks after beginning our work together, David told me he was "starting to find nicotine offensive." He was still smoking between ten and fifteen cigarettes a day, but a month earlier his daily intake had been twenty, so we were moving in the right direction. (Six months later, he was down to six cigarettes a day.)

It was clear to me by this time that the effects of David's treatment were holding, so we could see each other less often. I phased his frequency of visits back to twice monthly and later to once a month. The stress of midterm exams a few months later brought back some of David's pain and tension, and he returned to my office with significant muscle tension in the neck and upper back. Chiropractic adjustments similar to those I had used on the first visit once again brought swift relief.

His exam-week pain was more an aberration than a new pattern. In general, he sustained the progress apparent in the first two or three visits with rare interruptions.

Clyde Ford, D.C., in his thoroughly engaging book, *Where Healing Waters Meet: Touching Mind and Emotion Through the Body*, notes that there are many references in the medical literature on the healing effect of the mind on the body, but hardly any on the healing effect of the body on the mind. Dr. Ford arrived in the body-mind arena quite unexpectedly. While performing a routine first-visit exam on a patient with lower back pain, he was startled to find his patient shaking from head to toe, crying out in pain, totally out of proportion to the light touch used in the examination.

It turned out that the rotation of the patient's leg during the exam had triggered a long-suppressed memory of being raped by her father at age eleven. For the next twenty minutes, she cried as he held her hand. "I came to see you for my back," she said, "not for this." Ford offered to continue the exam the next day. Then, when she arose from the table, most of her pain was gone. To his great credit, Dr. Ford, rather than writing off the experience as an interesting anomaly and forgetting about it, embarked instead on a lengthy study of the history of therapeutic touch through the centuries. He developed a method he calls somatosynthesis, which aims to consciously utilize touch as part of the process for healing emotional wounds.

I have read many books by chiropractors, and none has touched me as deeply as *Where Healing Waters Meet*. If the chiropractic profession has a primary flaw (all professions do, I believe), it may be an overemphasis on physical causation of illness and a corresponding underemphasis on emotion and spirit. Clyde Ford's work moves us in the direction of healing this imbalance.

He is not alone in this, however. While the standard medical literature has little to say about the effect of bodywork on the healing of the mind, the subject has drawn increasing attention in recent years from practitioners and teachers of many natural healing arts. Some Western practitioners of traditional Chinese acupuncture, particularly those in the lineage of English acupuncturist Dr. J.R. Worsley, have been in the forefront of this movement. Dianne Connelly, Ph.D., M.Ac., co-founder of the Traditional Acupuncture Institute in Columbia, Maryland, provides both a theoretical framework and numerous case histories of body-mind interactions in her book *Traditional Acupuncture: The Law of the Five Elements*.

I have attended Dr. Connelly's talks, have been treated with traditional acupuncture, and have referred many patients to acupuncturists. I am particularly impressed by the way Chinese diagnosis of apparently physical ailments like back pain, bladder disorders, or premenstrual syndrome includes attention to the patient's emotional and mental patterns. Even more unusual is the way the patient's response to acupuncture is measured not solely by the disappearance of physical symptoms, but also by the depth of the overall energetic shift manifest in emotional no less than physical terms.

Edgar Cayce's health readings consistently recognize not only physical, but mental and spiritual components in all disease. Though the patient might have sought help for an ailment apparently physical in nature, Cayce consistently looked deeper, probing the meaning of the illness, pointing out causative factors in the patient's outlook on life, along with the physical causes. Similarly, Cayce always included physical measures like spinal manipulation and massage as part of the recommended therapy for what would be seen by conventional medicine as mental problems. From Cayce's vantage point, there was no such thing as a purely mental or purely physical condition.

Sources to which I've referred, from Edgar Cayce to Chinese medicine to the Ayurvedic system of India, agree that there are energy centers in the body which, among other attributes, act as points for the interface of body, mind, and spirit. The two systems of energy medicine with which I am most familiar, the Indian-derived polarity therapy system and the readings of Edgar Cayce, both postulate a series of seven energy centers.

On the physical level, each of these centers is correlated with a nerve plexus and an endocrine gland. In addition, they are considered to have a wide range of other correlations; each is believed to have a corresponding color, musical tone, element, focus of meaning, and more. I know of no way for science to either prove or disprove any of this. For now, it would probably be fair to consider it a traditional paradigm meriting further study.

While there are differences between the maps offered by Cayce and the Indian tradition, the areas of agreement predominate.

Chart 1
The Centers According to Edgar Cayce[3]

Center	Location	Color	Element	Meaning
1	Gonads	Red	Earth	Seeking Sustenance
2	Cells of Leydig	Orange	Water	Male/Female Balance
3	Adrenals	Yellow	Fire	Power/Self-Assertion
4	Thymus	Green	Air	Love
5	Thyroid	Blue	Ether	Will
6	Pineal	Indigo	—	Light/Seat of Soul
7	Pituitary	Violet	—	Oneness

Chart Two

The Centers According to Western
Interpreters of Indian Tradition[4]

Center	Location	Color	Element	Meaning
1	Base of Spine	Red	Earth	Basic Survival
2	Sacral Plexus	Orange	Water	Sexuality
3	Solar Plexus	Yellow	Fire	Power/Self-Assertion
4	Heart	Green	Air	Love
5	Throat	Blue	Ether	Creative Expression
6	Forehead	Indigo	—	Mind, Vision
7	Top of Head	Violet	—	Spirituality

Recall now that when David was in the midst of his break-through experience at our first visit, he saw vistas of blues and greens, "like a trail of lights . . . going up and down my back." From one point of view, this can be seen as a beautiful but mean-ingless set of signals within the nervous system.

But let's assume for a moment (please temporarily suspend disbelief if you need to) that it's more than a random set of nerve signals. From another point of view, it can be seen as an indica-tion of activity at the fourth (green) and fifth (blue) centers. And the correspondence doesn't stop there. When we look further, we see that David's primary areas of pain were in the upper back (fourth center) and neck (fifth center). His lung problems relate to the air element (fourth center), and one could make a credible case that he was working on issues of love (fourth) and will (fifth).

Is there value in looking at things from this standpoint? Maybe so. My speaking with David about it allowed him to view both his imbalance and his healing process from a broader perspective. For a student of psychology, philosophy, and religion, this was both stimulating and motivating. If I discuss energy centers with a patient, as I did with David after his intense experiences, I al-ways take care to note that this perspective is one of many

viewpoints from which the whole picture may be seen and inter-
preted. I want to engage the imagination, not create a new
orthodoxy.

In my opinion, no system possesses the sole accurate description of reality. Each contains a partial measure of the whole truth,
and each can add to our understanding of ourselves and our
world. In terms of allegiance to truth and respect for the individual, I strongly believe that no one should ever feel compelled
or pressured out of loyalty (to doctor, teacher, or anyone else) to
adopt one world view and reject all others. I don't limit myself in
this way, and I certainly don't want to convey such a limitation to
my patients or readers.

For me, the willingness to entertain different viewpoints at the
same time is a cornerstone of holism. In seeking to more fully
understand the whole person, we need the benefit of many
minds, many experiences, and many cultures, even when these
are in partial disagreement with each other. While this seems
paradoxical, it may be that turning knowledge into wisdom is a
fundamentally paradoxical process. What we lose in certainty, we
gain in understanding.

CHAPTER 7

A MOST UNUSUAL CASE

George, a thirty-year-old college student whom I saw in my first year of practice, taught me something about the power of chiropractic and the limitations of my own assumptions. More than a decade later, he remains among the most unusual cases I have ever encountered.

A year prior to my seeing him, George was in a motorcycle wreck and barely escaped with his life. Hit by a car on a highway, he was thrown thirty feet through the air. Though he miraculously fractured no bones other than those in his nose, he did have a concussion, a dislocated shoulder, and numerous strains and lacerations. He experienced a great deal of physical pain in many parts of his body during a month-long hospitalization. But within two months, he was free of pain.

There was, however, one persistent symptom with which none of his previous doctors had been able to help—constant nausea. "It's like I always want to throw up, especially after eating a meal," he said.

Treated by a series of doctors—an internist, a neurologist, a psychiatrist, and a homeopath—he showed no improvement. George was referred to me by the last of these, a medical physician who specialized in homeopathy (a healing art in which highly diluted substances are used as medicines). That doctor, seeing that his efforts on George's behalf were not working and knowing that virtually everything else had been tried, sent him to me on the chance that the problem was due to a spinal subluxation.

At our initial consultation, I queried George in depth about his diet. It turned out he had particular difficulty digesting protein foods, meats especially. This can be an indication that the stomach is producing insufficient quantities of hydrochloric acid, which breaks down proteins so that they may be digested and assimiliated.

As a chiropractor, I had two angles from which to approach this situation. A "relieve-the-symptoms" approach would dictate prescribing supplemental hydrochloric acid tablets with meals. These can be purchased at any health food store. If the body is not producing adequate hydrochloric acid, according to this line of reasoning, we should help it along by providing the missing ingredient from an external source.

A traditional chiropractic approach, on the other hand, asks, "Why is the body not producing enough hydrochloric acid?" The answer, in some cases, is that if there is inadequate nerve supply to the stomach, it will not be able to produce a normal amount of hydrochloric acid.

The nerve supply to the stomach comes from two areas: the fifth through ninth thoracic levels in the upper back (T5-9) and the first cervical level at the top of the neck. The T5-9 area may seem the logical suspect, since it is geographically closest to the stomach. But in George's case, it was that crucial first cervical that attracted my attention as I performed my first-visit examination.

When I tested the vertebrae of George's neck, pressing them to see if there were any abnormalities in movement, only one level seemed unusual—the top vertebra on the left side. I sent George for x-rays as a precautionary measure, to be certain the accident hadn't left residual damage I couldn't detect with a physical exam. Fortunately, the x-rays showed no unsuspected abnormalities, and the next day I adjusted the joint where the first cervical vertebra meets the occiput at the very top of the neck. I also recommended that he go to the health food store to pick up a bottle of hydrochloric tablets to take with his meals.

When George came back the following day, he had great news. "Doc, the nausea's gone, it's just totally out of here. I can't believe it! I sure hope this lasts," he said.

So did I. I assumed, beginner chiropractor that I was, that this was a symptomatic response to the hydrochloric acid tablets and wondered whether the effect would decrease with time. I needn't have worried. George had gotten lost on the way to the health food store and never purchased the tablets. Still disbelieving the evidence before my eyes, I asked him what he had been eating, wondering whether the nausea had disappeared in response to some dietary change.

A tall, friendly looking man with something of a potbelly, George explained a bit sheepishly that his entire dietary intake the day before had consisted of ice cream, pecans, and beer. These seemed to be mighty unlikely therapeutic agents, and I finally realized that there really was no further question—the adjustment of the first cervical vertebra had done the job.

George's nausea never returned in the four years we stayed in contact. I did, by the way, have some long talks with him about nutrition, particularly focusing on the need to have more vegetables and far less of the fats and alcohol he loved so much. I hoped he would take at least a few small steps in this direction, but he left for school two weeks after we started treatment. I remember thinking that I was like a gardener planting seeds. Some would bear fruit, and some wouldn't.

I next saw George two years later, when he needed help for some lower back pain. He had become a vegetarian and proudly announced that he was even making his own yogurt. From someone who used to subsist on bacon, eggs, beer, pizza, ice cream, and cola drinks (along with a few vegetables), this was music to my ears. He had also started to meditate and was practicing T'ai Chi and yoga. He looked better than ever and had a calmness about him that wasn't there the first time we met.

Seeing George again, three years into my practice, I for the first time had an inkling of what must be a familiar feeling to an older doctor who has stayed in the same community for many years. I saw that some seeds really do reach fruition and that you never really know the full effects of the work you do at the time you are doing it. I went home that day feeling like the older doctor, and I liked the feeling.

CHIROPRACTIC
AND
MANUAL MEDICINE

CHAPTER 8

CHIROPRACTIC: An ALTERNATIVE HEALING ART ENTERS THE MAINSTREAM

The movie *Lorenzo's Oil* offers a powerful illustration of the forces that have propelled the alternative health movement since its inception. In the movie, young Lorenzo's parents, faced with a severely ill child whose disease has no known medical cure, move heaven and earth (and a reluctant medical establishment) to save his life. Against all odds, they succeed.

The intensity of their refusal to accept things as they are and the way they demand of both themselves and others a willingness to explore unorthodox alternative healing methods are precisely the factors that have enabled chiropractic and other natural healing arts to survive and even thrive in the face of determined opposition from organized medicine.

In 1991, after well over a decade of litigation, the United States Supreme Court affirmed a lower court ruling declaring the American Medical Association et al. guilty of anti-trust violations that were part of an ongoing conspiracy to "contain and eliminate" (the AMA's own words) the chiropractic profession. As a result of the *Wilk v. AMA* suit, the medical profession reversed its longstanding ban on interprofessional cooperation between medical doctors and chiropractors, agreed to publish the full findings of the court in the *Journal of the American Medical Association*, and paid a large sum of money which is now being used for chiropractic research.

This has not undone the effects of a well-organized anti-chiropractic campaign by organized medicine (which at one point even included attempting to rig in advance a federally mandated study on chiropractic!),[1] but it certainly points to the dawning of a new day.

Chiropractic Research: Clinical Studies and the "Outcomes Revolution"

Spinal manual therapy, of which chiropractors are the primary providers, has now been shown by reputable researchers to be the most demonstrably effective healing method for the most common kinds of lower back pain. Each year brings the publication of more studies (published in both medical and chiropractic journals), gradually expanding the range of conditions for which chiropractic should be considered a treatment of choice.

This was not always so. For years, chiropractors were criticized for offering only anecdotal evidence (stories of people who got well under chiropractic care) in support of their methods. Despite the fact that only an estimated fifteen percent of orthodox medical interventions are validated by rigorous scientific research,[2] chiropractic was repeatedly attacked as unscientific, in contrast to the presumably altogether scientific medical profession.

Two things have changed. First, as you will see in this chapter, there is now a substantial body of chiropractic research, performed under accepted scientific protocols, which even the most die-hard skeptics cannot refute. Second, there has been an increased emphasis, largely driven by governmental and economic pressures, given to what is now called "outcomes research," which in part involves asking patients to rate their degree of pain relief, their return to proper function in daily activities, their satisfaction with treatment, and other related factors. Outcomes research has a strong subjective component, but has risen in stature because it has the overriding virtue of including what, after all, is the whole purpose of the healing arts—to bring improved health and relief from pain and suffering, *as judged by the patients themselves.*

The full effects of the outcomes research revolution are yet to be felt. But one thing is clear already: patients are growing very impatient with many orthodox medical therapies and are "voting with their feet." They are flocking in droves to alternative practitioners of all sorts,[3] some of whose approaches already have significant scientific validation (chiropractic being the most prominent example) and others whose methods have yet to face the scrutiny of rigorous research.

This trend, unprecedented in its magnitude and probably nowhere near the peak of the curve as yet, portends a significant realignment in the healing arts as we know them, probably within the next generation. While it is still possible that the forces of orthodoxy may wage temporarily successful rear-guard actions in some countries, blocking valid alternative methods from attaining equal status in terms of licensure and insurance reimbursement, it appears that a critical mass has already been reached and that major changes will continue at an accelerating pace.

The chiropractic profession is in the unusual—and perhaps unique—position of having one foot inside the establishment (with licensure, insurance reimbursement, accredited training institutions, and an increasingly broad scientific research base), while the other is firmly rooted in the alternative camp (with a philosophy of natural healing that in most cases relegates drug therapy to a position of last resort, rather than first).

As such, chiropractic provides a rare modern example of how a healing art, born in rebellion against the status quo, enters the mainstream. The history of chiropractic is for the most part an inspiring story of the triumph of the underdog, but it also contains a traveler's advisory as to the perils of the journey.

Historical Roots

Spinal manipulation has existed in one form or another for millennia. Accounts of manipulative therapies go as far back as 2700 B.C. in China, and a similar legacy has been bequeathed to us by ancient civilizations from Babylonia to Central America to Tibet.

Hippocrates (460 B.C.) was an early practitioner of spinal manipulation and, according to some scholars, the Father of Medicine used manipulation "not only to reposition vertebrae, but also thereby to cure a wide variety of dysfunctions."[4] The Hippocratic Corpus, recorded by physician-scholars in Alexandria, Egypt, when that city was the cultural center of Western civilization, includes detailed descriptions of manipulative methods.

Galen, a Greek-born Roman physician who lived in the second century A.D. and whose approach to healing set the officially recognized standard in Western medicine for 1,500 years after his death, also utilized spinal manipulation and reported successfully resolving a patient's hand weakness and numbness by manipulating the seventh cervical vertebra.[5]

As Europe endured what later would be known as the Dark Ages, these healing traditions were preserved in the learning centers of the Middle East by the ascendant Arabic civilization. Later, this body of knowledge returned to Europe, and the works of Hippocrates and Galen formed the foundation of Renaissance medicine. Ambroise Paré, sometimes called the Father of Surgery, used manipulation to treat French vineyard workers in the sixteenth century.[6]

During the centuries that followed, up to the beginning of the modern era, manipulative techniques were passed down from generation to generation within families. These "bone-setting" methods, which were transmitted not only from father to son but often from mother to daughter, played an important role in the history of nonmedical healing in Great Britain and similar methods are common in the folk medicine of many nations.

Birth of the Modern Professions

In the second half of the nineteenth century, the United States was a crucible of natural healing theory and practice. Two manipulation-based healing arts, osteopathy and chiropractic, trace their origins to that era. Both began in the American Midwest.

Neither emerged in a vacuum. A medical physician, Dr. J. Evans Riadore, wrote in 1843 in *Irritation of the Spinal Nerves* that "if any organ is deficiently supplied with nervous energy or of blood, its functions immediately, and sooner or later its structure, become deranged." Robert Leach, D.C., in *The Chiropractic Theories: A Synopsis of Scientific Research*, says of this, "Apparently Riadore concluded that irritation of the spinal nerve roots resulted in diseases; he even advised manipulation to treat this disorder."[7]

Dr. Riadore's work predated by decades the development of osteopathy by Andrew Taylor Still in the 1870s and the introduction of chiropractic by Daniel David Palmer in the 1890s. Whether or not Still and Palmer were personally aware of Riadore's work, and it seems likely that they were, their pioneering efforts certainly occurred in a context where work such as Riadore's was in the public domain.

Interestingly, Riadore's statement about deficiency of "nervous energy or of blood" summarizes in one phrase the respective founding principles of chiropractic and osteopathy. Since its beginnings, chiropractic has attributed the central role in health to the nervous system. Osteopathy is founded on the "Law of the Artery," with which Dr. Still asserted the primacy of the circulatory system.

Both Still and Palmer formulated their hypotheses and built their new professions against a backdrop of medical orthodoxy which they found to be frequently ineffective and sometimes barbaric. Dr. Still, a Missouri country doctor, had lost three of his children to spinal meningitis. The standard treatment of the era was cauterization (burning through the skin with a hot iron), followed by the application of bloodsucking leeches to the raw exposed tissues of the spinal area. After the death of his children, like the Biblical Job, Still cried out in his pain for understanding.

He spent the remainder of his life developing the natural healing art he called osteopathy.

Chiropractic: Then and Now

D.D. Palmer founded chiropractic on the premise that the vertebral subluxation was the cause of virtually all disease and the chiropractic adjustment its cure. This "one cause-one cure" philosophy has played a central role in chiropractic history—first as a guiding principle and later as an historical remnant, a bull's-eye at which the slings and arrows of organized medicine have repeatedly been hurled.

While few contemporary chiropractors would endorse such a simplistic formulation, it nonetheless remains true that the *raison d'être* of the chiropractic profession is the detection and correction of spinal subluxations. Chiropractors may, in fact, do much more, but it is our ability to do this one thing well that has allowed us to survive for a century under a constant barrage of medical opposition—some of it justified, most of it not.

The "one cause-one cure" adherents among the early chiropractors had two major political effects on the development of the profession. First, their deep faith in the truth of their message combined with the sometimes stunningly positive results of chiropractic adjustments created a strong and steadily growing activist constituency of chiropractic supporters. In their zeal, they forged a grassroots movement which assured the survival of the profession through some very stormy years in the first half of the twentieth century. But at the same time, by sometimes making inflated claims and failing to back these up with hard evidence, some early chiropractors also managed to convince most medical physicians and, through them, a substantial portion of the general public that chiropractors were not to be trusted.

In this conflict, the medical profession was by no means a disinterested party solely seeking to protect the public well-being. It faced in chiropractic an intrepid economic competitor with a competing philosophy that raised the possibility of healing without drugs, which were—and still are—the medical profession's primary healing tool.

The *Wilk v. AMA* suit brought to light a decades-long pattern of political intrigue which exposed the AMA for what it was: a trade association whose principal loyalty was to the self-interest of its membership. Fortunately in the United States antitrust laws make it illegal for one profession to try to destroy another. The American judicial system may sometimes seem to move interminably slowly, but in this case justice finally prevailed.

A Complex Legacy

Contemporary chiropractors have inherited both the positive and negative aspects of this complex legacy. We look back at our professional forebears and honor the level of sacrifice their commitment called forth, while at the same time seeking to adapt to the needs of a new era.

Our task is in many ways easier than theirs. Starting with D.D. Palmer, thousands of chiropractors were charged with practicing medicine without a license. Hundreds, including Palmer himself, went to jail.[8] Civil disobedience was an integral part of the early development of the chiropractic profession, as it would later become in the civil rights movement. When Dr. Palmer was jailed in 1906, he said, "I have never considered it beneath my dignity to do anything to relieve human suffering." Like Henry David Thoreau before him and Martin Luther King, Jr., later, Palmer understood that the defense of basic rights sometimes requires time behind bars.

Because of the sacrifices made by Palmer and so many others through the years, chiropractors today are able to practice freely, and the profession is truly coming of age in our time. Over the past several decades, the chiropractic profession has undergone profound changes, as standards in education, research, and practice methodology have steadily risen to meet the demands of a fast-changing society. An excellent historical review, for those seeking greater detail, is contained in the book, *Dynamic Chiropractic Today,* written by a former president of the British Chiropractors Association, Michael Copland-Griffiths, D.C.

Chiropractors are now licensed throughout the English-speaking world and in many other nations as well. Educational standards and testing procedures are rigorous. Numerous college science courses are required prior to entering chiropractic school, and the chiropractic college curriculum extends four or more years. Highly trained faculty fill both the basic science and clinical science departments at all chiropractic colleges, which are accredited by government-supervised agencies in the various countries.

In Australia, the first wholly government-funded chiropractic training program in the world was incorporated into a university curriculum in 1980. In Quebec, a similar program began in 1993 at the state (provincial) university. These programs are a sign of things to come and foreshadow a far greater integration of chiropractic into the health care system of the future.

The greatest strides in the late twentieth century have been in the area of research. No longer can chiropractors be criticized for lacking a firm base of scientific research. The tide has truly turned, as chiropractic has entered the modern era.

Chiropractic Research

The early leaders of the chiropractic profession recognized the value of research. Dr. B.J. Palmer, the founder's son, conducted numerous studies between the 1910s and the 1950s, documenting the effects of chiropractic adjustments on such physical functions as blood pressure, heart rate, respiration, and brainwave patterns.

Unfortunately, B.J. Palmer's studies, like other chiropractic (and medical) research from the first half of the twentieth century, do not meet the criteria demanded by the modern scientific community. In the context of their time, however, an era when medical clinical trials were just beginning, Palmer's work marked the first serious attempt at objective measurement of the physiological effects of the chiropractic adjustment.

Through the years of Palmer's preeminence in the chiropractic world, many other independent chiropractors and chiropractic colleges also carried the torch of research, exploring new adjusting methods and measuring their effects. Like Palmer's studies, these, too, are of significant historical interest, but did not follow the rigorous scientific protocols demanded of today's research.

By the early 1970s, the scientific gap between chiropractic and medicine had widened, and the more far-sighted chiropractic leaders realized that it had to be closed as quickly as possible. Looking back now from the vantage point of the 1990s, it is remarkable that so much has been accomplished in such a short time.

Dr. Suh and the University of Colorado Project

Beginning in the 1970s, first with grants from the International Chiropractors Association and later with added financial support from the American Chiropractic Association and the federal government of the United States, Chung Ha Suh, Ph.D., and his colleagues at the Biomechanics Department of the University of Colorado began a series of studies which have provided an extensive body of chiropractic-related scientific research.

It is worth noting that Dr. Suh, the first American college professor willing to stick his neck out for chiropractic research, grew up in Korea, where he had not been subjected to the same lifelong anti-chiropractic bias as his American colleagues. In undertaking this research, he had to withstand intense pressure from powerful forces within the American medical and academic establishments. The AMA and cohorts condemned chiropractic for lack of scientific underpinning, while at the same time doing everything in their considerable power to prevent chiropractors from ever obtaining the funding and university connections necessary for the development of such a research base.

Time and again in American history, it has been immigrants who have brought to our land the fresh perspectives needed to move our society forward. In addition, progress has often required the courage to stand up against politically powerful forces of stagnation. Dr. C.H. Suh stands as a modern exemplar of both these traditions.

The research at the University of Colorado involved two major projects. In one, Dr. Suh developed a complex computer model of the cervical spine, which allowed a deeper understanding of spinal joint mechanics and their relationship to the chiropractic adjustment.

The second project involved studying the effects of compression on spinal nerve roots. Seth Sharpless, Ph.D.; Marvin Luttges, Ph.D.; and their colleagues demonstrated that minuscule amounts of pressure on a nerve root (10mm Hg, equal to a feather falling on your hand), resulted in up to a fifty percent decrease in electrical transmission down the course of the nerve supplied by that root.[9] Chiropractors have long claimed that minimal pressure on nerves could have a significant physiological impact. This study gave credence to such claims and offered a promising path for future research.

Most of the recent interdisciplinary clinical research jointly conducted by chiropractors and medical physicians has been done outside the United States, which still remains the last, strongest bastion of the medical *ancien régime*. The most influential research studies of the past decade were done in Canada, Great Britain, and the Netherlands.

The Canadian Study

In 1985, a landmark study was published in the *Canadian Family Physician*[10] which researched the effects of chiropractic adjustments for people with severe and chronic lower back pain. The approximately 300 subjects in this study had been "totally disabled" by back pain for an average of seven years and had gone through the full gamut of standard medical interventions.

The study found that after two to three weeks of daily chiropractic adjustments, between seventy-nine and ninety-three percent of those patients without spinal stenosis (narrowed spinal cord) had good to excellent results, reporting substantially decreased pain and increased mobility. Even among those with a congenitally or developmentally narrowed spinal cord, a significant number showed substantial improvement. Remember that every single one of these people had gone through extensive, unsuccessful medical treatment prior to being allowed to participate as a research subject. After chiropractic treatment, over seventy percent of those studied were improved to the point of having no work restrictions. Moreover, follow-up a year later demonstrated that the changes were long-lasting.

These results are remarkable, but what was extraordinary about the Canadian study was the fact that it was jointly administered by Dr. J.R. Cassidy, a chiropractor, and Dr. W.H. Kirkaldy-Willis, a world-renowned orthopedic surgeon. In 1993, Dr. Cassidy became the first chiropractor to be named research director of a university orthopedics department—at the University of Saskatchewan, where this research was done.

The landmark Canadian study clearly demonstrates the effectiveness of chiropractic adjustments for treating chronic lower back pain, even when standard medical interventions have been exhausted. Yet, sadly, many physicians seem unaware of this study—and too few take the logical next step of referring patients with these symptoms to a chiropractor.

The British Study

In 1990, the *British Medical Journal* published a study called "Low Back Pain of Mechanical Origin: Randomised Comparison of Chiropractic and Hospital Outpatient Treatment," by an orthopedic surgeon, Dr. Thomas Meade.[11] Meade's research compared chiropractic manipulation with standard hospital outpatient treatment for lower back pain. The medical treatment consisted of wearing a corset and attending physical therapy sessions. Over 700 patients were involved in the study.

Dr. Meade concluded:

"For patients with low-back pain in whom manipulation is not contraindicated, chiropractic almost certainly confers worthwhile, long-term benefit in comparison to hospital outpatient management."

In a later interview on a Canadian Broadcasting Corporation program, Dr. Meade said:

"Our trial showed that chiropractic is a very effective treatment, *more effective than conventional hospital outpatient treatment for low-back pain* [emphasis added], particularly in patients who had back pain in the past and

who [developed] severe problems. So, in other words, it is
most effective in precisely the group of patients that you
would like to be able to treat ... One of the unexpected findings was that the treatment difference—the benefit of
chiropractic over hospital treatment—actually persists for
the whole of that three-year period [of the study] ... it looks
as though the treatment that the chiropractors give does
something that results in a very long-term benefit."[12]

The major significance of the Meade study is that it is the first
randomized study to demonstrate long-term benefits from
chiropractic care. One baseless, but persistent, criticism of
chiropractic has been that while it may offer short-term relief, it
is of no lasting value. The Canadian and British studies, taken
together, should by any reasonable standard be sufficient to lay
this old falsehood to rest. Nonetheless, the criticism continues to
appear in print and needs to be answered forthrightly whenever
it rears its head.

The RAND Study

In 1992, the widely respected RAND Corporation, a health-
care think tank, released a study on the appropriateness of spinal
manipulation for lower back pain. Authored by a
multidisciplinary panel headed by Paul Shekelle, M.D., the study
marked the first time that representatives of this prestigious
group had officially recognized spinal manipulation as an appropriate treatment for some patients with lower back pain. RAND's
procedures involved an extensive review of the scientific literature on the treatment of back pain and a consensus process
among the participants to determine areas of agreement.

The rather limited nature of RAND's endorsement of spinal
manipulation must be seen in context to be properly understood.
RAND is known for its thoroughgoing critical evaluations and the
great caution of its assessments, which is part of the reason that
its conclusions are often taken by federal officials as something
close to the final word on health matters. While its conclusions
on spinal manipulation failed to go as far as many chiropractors

would have liked, they nonetheless were far more favorable than RAND's recent pronouncements on other controversial medical issues such as heart surgery.

The national media were quick to grasp the significance of the RAND report. In the weeks and months immediately following its release, high-profile news reports appeared in American newspapers, magazines, and electronic media, declaring that chiropractic was finally being "accepted." Of course, millions of chiropractic patients had already accepted it happily for years, but the RAND report marked the scaling of an inner wall of the health establishment.

The Dutch Study

A Dutch study published in the *British Medical Journal* in 1992 compared the results of back and neck pain patients treated with physical therapy against those given chiropractic manipulation and also compared these two methods to placebo treatment and standard medical treatment by a general practitioner.

The results were impressive and showed that both chiropractic manipulation and physical therapy were significantly more effective than a placebo treatment or treatment by a general practitioner. In addition, those receiving manipulation showed more improvement than the physical therapy patients, in fewer visits.[13]

Additional Studies

• An Australian study showed that patients who were treated by chiropractors lost four times fewer work days from low-back pain than those treated by medical doctors.[14]

• A cost-comparison study in the *Journal of Occupational Medicine* demonstrated that the compensation costs for lost work time were ten times as high for those receiving standard, nonsurgical medical care than for those who were treated by chiropractors.[15]

• A study of Florida workers' compensation cases indicated that patients receiving chiropractic care were temporarily disabled for half the length of time, were hospitalized at less than half the rate, and accrued bills less than half as high as patients receiving medical care for similar conditions.[16]

• Preliminary results of a study on headaches showed spinal manipulation to be more effective than prescription medication for long-term pain relief. The chiropractic patients maintained their levels of improvement, while those treated with medication returned to their pretreatment status in an average of four weeks after completion of treatment.[17]

• The North American Spine Society (an interdisciplinary body consisting of expert practitioners and academics from the medical, osteopathic, and chiropractic professions) rated spinal manipulative therapy in Category I, the highest rating, for treatment of lower back pain. Chiropractic adjustments were described as generally accepted, well-established, and widely used.[18]

• AV MED, the largest health maintenance organization (HMO) in the southeastern United States, sent 100 medically unresponsive patients to a chiropractor. Eighty-six percent of this group were helped. As a result of two to three weeks of chiropractic care, all twelve patients medically diagnosed as needing disc surgery were able to avoid surgery, saving AV MED $250,000 and sparing the patients the risks and consequences of unnecessary surgery.[19]

• A study published in the *Western Journal of Medicine* in 1989 found that chiropractic patients were more satisfied with their care than back pain patients of family practice physicians by a ratio of three to one. Interestingly, initial discussion of this study in medical journals generally assumed that the greater satisfaction rates among chiropractic patients were due entirely to allegedly superior doctor-patient relationships on the part of chiropractors. Left out of the analysis for the most part was the possibility that the difference may have been due in large measure to the greater effectiveness of chiropractic treatment methods.[20]

In fact, chiropractic manipulation has been shown to be far more effective than the bed rest and prescription medications routinely prescribed by family practice physicians and general practitioners for back and neck pain, as shown in the study that follows.

- A clinical trial found that bed rest plus nonsteroidal anti-inflammatory medication (which together form the standard method with which family practice physicians and general practitioners treat low back pain) *brought results worse than a placebo treatment.*[21] This is particularly problematic in light of the fact that more people initially go to these primary care doctors for low back pain than to any other type of practitioner. Chiropractic treatment for lower back pain has been shown in many studies to be significantly superior to a placebo, and no reputable study has ever shown it to be worse than a placebo.

- The November 1992 issue of the *Journal of Family Practice*, the major journal for family practice physicians in the United States, included three strongly pro-chiropractic articles, which urged readers to "reevaluate chiropractic" and "reconsider referrals to chiropractors for musculoskeletal problems." The first paper was co-authored by Peter Curtis, M.D., of the Department of Family Medicine at the University of North Carolina, Chapel Hill, and Geoffrey Bove, D.C., a Ph.D. candidate in the Department of Cell Biology and Anatomy at the same school. The other two articles were editorials supporting the Curtis-Bove article, one by noted researcher Daniel Cherkin, Ph.D., and the other by three Israeli medical doctors who supported the conclusions of Drs. Curtis and Bove.[22]

- A study by the Gallup Organization determined that ninety percent of chiropractic patients rated their treatment as effective, and eighty percent were satisfied with the treatment they received and felt that most of their expectations were met.[23]

Chiropractors and the millions who have benefited from chiropractic care over the years believed all of this to be true from the beginning. That's why they fought so hard for its full acceptance as a legitimate, recognized healing art. Finally, enough objective scientific data now exists to show that their faith in chiropractic was not misplaced.

As scientific research continues to validate the chiropractic approach, the case for full recognition and integration grows stronger year by year. This is the path required of all alternative healing methods seeking to cross the bridge from alternative to mainstream. As each alternative enters the mainstream, the stream itself is forever changed.

CHAPTER 9

FOUNDATIONS OF THE CHIROPRACTIC MODEL

We have now seen a wealth of studies demonstrating that spinal manipulation is effective, but it is quite another matter to fully understand how and why. The search for an explanation has absorbed the attention of chiropractors since D.D. Palmer founded the profession in 1895.

The history of chiropractic, like all healing arts, is largely one in which empirical process has preceded theoretical formulation. In other words, from the earliest days practitioners have applied new manual treatment methods on an intuitive, empirical basis, noted that some are more effective than others, and theorized on the basis of these findings as to the underlying mechanisms.

When certain methods have demonstrated their effectiveness over a period of time, they, along with the theories used to explain them, become part of what we might call the "chiropractic corpus," the body of tradition, evidence, and practice which is the contribution of the chiropractic school of knowledge to the healing arts as a whole.

Not until the late twentieth century was this accumulated body of chiropractic knowledge sufficiently grounded in scientific research to allow wide recognition across professional boundaries. Fortunately, that point has now been reached. It, therefore, seems timely to review the nature of the chiropractic diagnostic and therapeutic model, so that it can be well understood by the public and other health professionals.

Part of this review is an examination of chiropractic theory past and present. It is important to sift out ideas which may have been state of the art in 1910 or 1950, but which are no longer fully tenable. Chief among these is the idea that the chiropractic adjustment works primarily by physically moving a vertebra that is out of place back into place.

The Bone-Out-of-Place Theory

The early chiropractors assumed that their adjustments worked by moving misaligned vertebrae back into line, thereby relieving pressure caused when those bones impinged directly on spinal nerves. The standard explanation given to patients was the analogy of stepping on a garden hose—if you step on the hose, the water can't get through, and then if you lift your foot off the hose, the free flow of water is restored. Similarly, the explanation went, the chiropractic adjustment removes the pressure of bone on nerve, thus allowing free flow of nerve impulses.

Based on the information available in the early years, such a theory was plausible. Chiropractors were able to feel interruptions in the symmetry of the spinal column with their well-trained hands and in many cases could verify this on x-ray (discovered in 1895, the same year as chiropractic). They would then adjust the vertebra with manual pressure, attempting to move it back into line. More often than not, patients reported significant functional improvements and healing effects.

But there are problems with the theory. This can most simply and directly be illustrated by noting the fact that, after an adjustment resulting in dramatic relief from headaches or sciatica, an x-ray will rarely show any discernible change in alignment. (Such comparative x-rays are now considered inappropriate, because of the unnecessary radiation exposure.) Long-term positive health changes have not been definitively shown to correlate with symmetrical alignment of spinal bones on any consistent basis.

Though much excellent work has been done by chiropractors whose understanding of their healing art was based on the bone-out-of-place theory, the theory has not stood the test of time. This does not mean that chiropractic is invalid, only that this late nineteenth-century explanation has been overtaken by newer developments.

While misalignments may play a role in the interpretation of spinal subluxations, they are no longer believed to play the central role. But if the old explanation of misaligned bones pressing on nerves is inadequate, what new theory has replaced it? To answer this question, we need to move beyond the essentially two-dimensional viewpoint of the misalignment theory and include motion as an added dimension.

The Intervertebral Motion Theory

In the 1930s, Belgian chiropractor Henri Gillet developed a theory of intervertebral motion and fixation, in which he asserted that it was loss of normal spinal joint movement, rather than misalignment, that was the underlying explanation for the vertebral subluxation. He agreed with the bone-out-of-place adherents that the interplay between the skeletal system and the nervous system was crucial, but parted ways with them regarding the causal process underlying the abnormal nerve signaling. Rather than attributing the subluxation's effects to direct pressure of misaligned bone on nerve, Gillet theorized that loss of proper joint dynamics was the underlying issue.

Later work by medical researchers Schmorl and Junghans, and many more who followed, verified the complex role of the "vertebral motor unit," consisting of bones, muscles, ligaments, blood vessels, and nerves. This model is now widely accepted.

All of these structural components are involved in the subluxation complex. Bypassing the old argument of whether the causative factor in the vertebral subluxation is the bone or the muscle, the work of Gillet, Schmorl, Junghans, and others allowed the problem to be seen from a broader, multifaceted perspective, in which all components of the intervertebral joint are involved in an elaborate interplay. This model first achieved profession-wide attention among chiropractors in the 1980s and now enjoys broad acceptance in chiropractic college curricula throughout the world.[1]

Jerome McAndrews, D.C., an early advocate of motion theory and practice who later served as president of Palmer College of Chiropractic, translated this model into visual terms when I spoke with him during preparation of this book:

> "View it as a mobile hanging from the ceiling. As it hangs there, it is in a state of dynamic equilibrium. Then, if you cut one of the strings, the whole mobile starts moving, because its balance has been upset. Eventually, it slows down and reaches a new state of dynamic equilibrium."

The body's musculoskeletal system works in much the same way, Dr. McAndrews explained. If its normal balance is disrupted, it has no choice but to compensate. Structural patterns will be altered to a greater or lesser degree, depending on the nature and intensity of the forces that threw off the old pattern of balance.

If chiropractic care is sought early, relatively little treatment may be required, because these compensations will not have had time to deeply imbed themselves structurally. Thus, a child injured playing football at age ten might need just one or two adjustments, but if that child waits until age forty before seeking chiropractic care (not an uncommon occurrence), the situation may prove far more complex. Patterns of long-term muscular rigidity, calcium deposits in ligaments, and significant structural shifts of the vertebral column or rib cage, for example, may set in with relative permanence.

In some such circumstances, when much time has passed, the achievable therapeutic goal may be limited to partial restoration of mobility and function. Returning to the once-upon-a-time perfection of the ten-year-old's pre-injury body becomes impossible somewhere along the way.

The theory of dynamic equilibrium, with its emphasis on intervertebral motion and fixation, has the great advantage of allowing, for the first time, a coherent explanation of chiropractic and the subluxation complex that can be communicated in familiar terms to medical practitioners and researchers. This has resulted in clearer lines of communication between chiropractors and medical professionals. While some hold onto the old model and terminology, the stage has been set for completion of this significant shift in perspective, as the new generation of chiropractic and medical practitioners who were trained after it took hold comes of age.

Wide-Ranging Effects of Spinal Manipulation

Restoring mobility to a joint by manipulation eases the stress at that joint and in the surrounding tissues. Unless complicating factors are present, muscular tension eases in the area that has been adjusted. As joint dysfunction decreases, other secondary symptoms such as pain, tingling, or numbness along the path of the nerves originating at the involved spinal level also improve.

Though the vast majority of chiropractic patients arrive seeking help for musculoskeletal problems like back pain, neck pain, and headaches, spinal adjustments can also have positive effects on other organs and systems. While chiropractic adjustments are directed to restoring motion at specific vertebral joints, the effects of these adjustments extend beyond the local area where the adjustive force is applied. Effects can extend to all structures served by the nerves originating in the spine.

Thus, neck adjustments can affect not only the neck and arms, but also the function of various organs in the head (via sympathetic pathways) and in the chest and upper abdomen (via the parasympathetic vagus nerve). Upper back adjustments can affect not only the upper back, but also organs in the chest and parts of the digestive tract. Adjustments of the lower back may influence not only the lower back and legs, but also the kidneys, pelvic organs, and lower digestive tract.

The First Chiropractic Adjustment:
A Case of Hearing Restored

The first chiropractic adjustment in 1895 was one in which the patient sought help for back pain and got results far beyond his expectations. Harvey Lillard, a deaf janitor in the building where D.D. Palmer had an office, came to Palmer bent over with back pain. Palmer gave him a spinal adjustment, after which Mr. Lillard stood up straight, was free of back pain, and able to hear for the first time in many years.

At first, it appeared that Palmer might have discovered a cure for deafness, but similar results were not forthcoming when other deaf people learned about Harvey Lillard and sought Palmer's help. And while there have been other instances through the years of hearing restored through spinal manipulation (including one by Canadian orthopedist J.F. Bourdillion, M.D.),[2] these have been rare, and no predictable pattern has emerged. The story of Lillard's recovery has been used for many years to disparage chiropractic, with repeated charges by the naysayers (primarily anti-chiropractic MDs) that such an event is impossible, because no spinal nerves supply the ear. Once, when I was testifying as an expert witness in a patient's automobile accident case, the opposing attorney, his voice dripping with sarcasm, attacked me with this very story.

It is important to refute the charge specifically. The underlying physiological mechanism is called the somato-autonomic reflex, fully recognized in all modern medical and chiropractic textbooks. Its name describes the interaction between the muscular and skeletal system (soma or body) and the autonomic (involuntary) portion of the nervous system. Signals initiated by spinal manipulation are transmitted via autonomic pathways to internal organs.

In the case of Palmer's first adjustment, the relevant nerve pathway starts in the upper back, coursing up the neck and into the skull along the sympathetic nerves which eventually lead to the blood vessels in the ear. Proper functioning of the hearing apparatus depends on a normal blood supply, which in turn depends on an adequate nerve supply.

While it is true that there are no *spinal* nerves as such directly supplying the ear, it is absolutely untrue that no nerve pathway links the two areas. The pathway exists, and any claims to the contrary betray ignorance of fully accepted modern physiology research.

Further Examples of Manipulation's Effects on Internal Organs

Just as there are autonomic pathways supplying the ear, similar pathways lead from the spine to all parts of the body. Research has verified that these pathways exist and that in some instances spinal manipulation can positively affect problems caused by them. The work of Czech neurologist Karel Lewit, M.D., American orthopedic surgeon John McMillan Mennell, M.D., and others has been particularly helpful in spreading these concepts beyond the chiropractic community. Dr. Lewit has for many years successfully used spinal manipulation to treat tonsillitis, breathing problems, migraine, vertigo, and much more.[3]

An example of a potential future direction for joint medical-chiropractic research is found in the book, *Chiropractic: Interprofessional Research*, a summary of research presented at the World Chiropractic Conference held in Venice, Italy, in 1982. A series of studies by chiropractors, working in concert with Italian medical doctors, demonstrated promising effects of chiropractic treatment in cases of vertigo, tinnitus (ringing in the ears), headaches, and visual disorders.[4]

There is far less research available concerning chiropractic's effects on visceral (internal organ) disorders than exists in relation to lower back pain and other musculoskeletal problems. This is because the chiropractic profession has had to prioritize the research it could afford to pursue in the absence of significant government funding. Proving the validity of chiropractic manipulation for those conditions most commonly treated by chiropractors (low back pain, neck pain, and headaches) has been the highest priority.

There is, nevertheless, a growing body of literature, some of it published in peer-reviewed scientific journals, on the effects of manipulation for problems related to internal organ dysfunction. Some of these are controlled clinical trials, while others are thought-provoking case studies which point to the need for more extensive future research.

Studies include:
- A randomized, controlled clinical study demonstrated that diastolic and systolic blood pressure decreased significantly in response to chiropractic adjustments of the thoracic spine (T1-T5), while placebo and control groups showed no such change. This study demonstrated short-term effects of manipulation on blood pressure and indicates a need for studies on long-term effects.[5]
- As noted earlier in this book, there have been two controlled clinical trials which studied the effects of spinal manipulation on dysmenorrhea. The results were quite promising, and further research is in progress.[6,7]
- A study at the National College of Chiropractic showed a marked increase in the activity levels of certain immune-system cells (PMNs and monocytes) after thoracic spine manipulation. These increases were significantly higher than in control groups, who were given either sham manipulation or soft-tissue manipulation.[8]
- A study involving seventy-three Danish chiropractors in fifty clinics showed satisfactory results in ninety-four percent of cases of infant colic. The results occurred within two weeks and involved an average of three treatments.[9]
- Several case studies have indicated that bladder dysfunction can be responsive to lower back manipulation.[10,11]
- Lung volume and forced vital capacity (a measure of lung strength) were shown in a series of cases to increase after chiropractic adjustments.[12,13]
- A seven-month-old infant suffering from chronic constipation since birth (with a history of hard, pellet-like stools following hours of painful straining) was restored to normal bowel function by full-spine and cranial adjustments.[14]
- A two-year-old child medically diagnosed with asthma and enuresis (bedwetting) improved dramatically as a result of spinal

adjustments, after medication had proved inadequate.[15]

• Pelvic pain and pelvic organ dysfunction, in which there was no accompanying lower back pain, was shown in a case study to resolve fully with chiropractic manipulation of the lumbar spine, after numerous failed attempts at treating the symptoms medically.[16]

• A five-year-old girl, who was experiencing up to seventy seizures a day, was treated with upper neck adjustments and became virtually seizure-free.[17]

Further exploration of chiropractic's effects on internal organ problems holds great promise. Studies are under way as this book goes to press, and many more are expected. This may turn out to be the most fertile area for chiropractic research in the twenty-first century.

The Chiropractic Perspective

Looking back over the material covered so far, how would the differences between the chiropractic approach and the standard medical model best be summarized?

First and foremost, the chiropractic model views symptoms in a broad context of health and body balance, not as isolated aberrations to be suppressed and then forgotten. Chiropractors recognize the need for thorough evaluation of symptoms, but do not assume that the elimination of symptoms is the ultimate goal of treatment. Just as peace is not the absence of war, health is not the absence of disease symptoms. The true goal is sustainable balance. This is recognized by chiropractors and by holistic medical physicians as well.

While chiropractors are trained in state-of-the-art diagnostic techniques and while chiropractic examination procedures overlap significantly with those used by conventional medical physicians, chiropractors evaluate the information gleaned from these methods from a perspective that recognizes the intricate structural and functional interplay among different parts of the body.

The contrasting medical and chiropractic diagnostic approaches to pain provide a case in point. In my experience, conventional medical physicians far more frequently than chiropractors make the assumption that the location of a pain is the location of its cause. Thus, knee pain is generally assumed to be a knee problem, shoulder pain is assumed to be a shoulder problem, and so forth. This pain-centered diagnostic logic frequently leads to increasingly sophisticated and invasive diagnostic and therapeutic procedures. (If physical examination of the knee fails to clearly define the problem, then the knee is x-rayed. If the x-ray fails to offer adequate clarification, then an MRI of the knee is performed, and so forth.)

Chiropractors also utilize these diagnostic tools. I refer some patients for x-rays and MRI studies. My point is not to criticize these methods, but to present an alternative diagnostic model. I have seen more than a few cases of knee trouble where this entire high-tech diagnostic scenario was played out, and the cause of the problem turned out to be in the lower back.

If the lower back is mechanically dysfunctional and in need of spinal manipulation, this can often place unusual stress on the knees. In cases of this sort, one can spend months or years medicating the knee symptoms with painkiller pills and/or steroid injections—or perform knee surgery—without ever addressing the real problem. *This is not an isolated hypothetical instance. It happens far too often.*

Whole-Body Context

The chiropractic approach to musculoskeletal pain involves evaluating the site of pain in a whole-body context. Shoulder, elbow, and wrist problems can, of course, be caused by problems in the shoulder, elbow, and wrist—but pain in all of these joints frequently has its source in the neck. Similarly, pain in the hip, knee, and ankle can also have its source at the site of the pain—but in many cases the source lies in the lower back. The need to consider this chain of causation is built into the core of chiropractic training.

Chiropractors from D.D. Palmer onward have purposely refrained from assuming that the site of a symptom is the site of its cause. They have assumed instead that *the source of the pain should be sought somewhere along the path of the nerves leading to and from the site of the symptoms.*

Thus, a pain in the knee might come from the knee itself, but if we trace the nerve pathways between the knee and the spine, we find along the way possible areas of causation in or around the hip, in the deep muscles of the buttocks or pelvis, in the sacroiliac joints, or in the lower spine.

Furthermore, if an imbalance does exist in the lower spine (at the fourth lumbar level, for example), it might have its source right there at L4 or might in turn be a compensation for another joint dysfunction elsewhere in the spine, perhaps in the middle or upper back. Thus, an integrated, whole-body approach to structure and function is of great value.

For a patient with an internal organ problem, chiropractic diagnostic logic would include evaluation of those spinal levels which are the source of the nerve supply to the involved area, as well as consideration of possible nutritional, environmental, and psychological causes. Chiropractic practice standards also mandate timely referral to a medical physician for diagnosis and/or treatment, for any condition that is acute and dangerous or when a reasonable trial of chiropractic treatment (current standards in most cases limit this to about one month) fails to bring satisfactory results.

Wellness and the Chiropractic Model

The chiropractic model pays heed to patients' nutritional needs, exercise habits, work conditions, and psychological health. In many cases, particularly with regard to nutrition and exercise, the chiropractor will act as a teacher, directly counseling patients on proper diet or exercise methods. In other instances, chiropractors will make referrals to other health practitioners or to appropriate classes in the community.

The traditional chiropractic philosophy I learned during my training anticipated in many respects the concepts that comprise the modern wellness paradigm. Aside from being taught the importance of good diet, exercise, and emotional health, we also learned that it is far better to practice prevention than to engage in crisis-care and that health is far more than the absence of symptoms. These ideas together form a respectable foundation for a profession that seeks to practice holism.

CHAPTER 10

EDGAR CAYCE'S HOLISTIC THEORIES ON MANUAL MEDICINE

A Perspective on Early Chiropractic and Osteopathy, with Potential Contemporary Applications

In the 1980s, when the *Journal of the American Medical Association (JAMA)* published its first editorial on holism, it traced the origin of the modern holistic health movement to the birth of Edgar Cayce in Hopkinsville, Kentucky, in 1877. I doubt that the *JAMA* editorial board intended this as a compliment to either Cayce or the holistic movement, but I believe the statement represents an accurate judgment.

The Cayce readings present an understandable, comprehensive view of health that recognizes body, mind, and spirit as co-equal fundamental building blocks. The readings embody a rare blend of vision and pragmatism, calling into play an inspired level of interaction among the will and aspirations of the individual, the workings of the physical body, and the forces of nature. For me, they are as uplifting and informative now as when I first came upon them. I find them accessible at deeper and deeper levels, the more experienced I become as a chiropractor and healing arts practitioner.

Cayce's theories on manual medicine are best understood in the context of his holistic overview. In the chapters that follow, I include Cayce's material on diet, exercise, meditation, visualization, and prayer, comparing and contrasting it with other sources. While the Cayce material no longer stands alone in its comprehensive sweep, I believe it is the most advanced Western synthesis of its time and perhaps of ours as well.

When we speak of an emerging holistic paradigm, it is not so much that the paradigm itself is new and therefore emergent, but rather that it has taken until now for it to begin blossoming fully on a broad scale in the West. The Chinese, Indians, and other Eastern and indigenous cultures the world over understood long ago that body, mind, and spirit are one. They never divided them in the first place. Their ancient healing arts are holistic in the deepest sense.

Edgar Cayce's unique contribution lies in articulating a holistic world view for the West, in language understandable to North Americans and Europeans. The fact that his material came through psychic methods undoubtedly prejudices some people against it from the start, but it has nonetheless achieved remarkably widespread attention and influence.

Many of the doctors who founded and developed the American Holistic Medical Association (AHMA), which now represents holistic medical doctors nationwide, were first introduced to holism through the Edgar Cayce readings or were strongly influenced by Cayce. Founding AHMA president Norman Shealy, M.D., and former president Gladys McGarey, M.D., are longtime proponents of Cayce holism.

The fact that Cayce's health information came through an individual in a non-ordinary state of awareness does not, in and of itself, mean that it is either valid or invalid. It deserves to be subjected to reasonable scrutiny and evaluated on its merits, just like any other system or theory. Furthermore, the Cayce material is probably not unique in its "altered state" origins. Legend has it that at least parts of Indian Ayurveda and traditional Chinese medicine sprang from individuals in similarly inspired states.

Cayce and Manual Medicine

As other parts of this book make clear, I have found Edgar Cayce's theories on many aspects of health and healing to be thought-provoking. They were what attracted me to chiropractic in the first place. I find his ideas on the interrelationships among spinal manipulation, the nervous system, and the circulatory system particularly intriguing.

I should state from the outset that, while Cayce's concepts draw on much well-accepted information on anatomy and physiology, few of the methods he speaks of have been well-researched in the modern era. The research that has been done is largely found in the osteopathic literature. I present Cayce's work as a theory worthy of consideration.

One question that often arises with regard to the Cayce readings is whether the principles and practices mentioned there are best represented by contemporary osteopathy or chiropractic. In my judgment, the real answer is neither. The closest analog to the Cayce readings is the osteopathy of the early twentieth century, and practitioners utilizing those methods are now few and far between.

Some things progress with the passage of time, but modernity is not always synonymous with advancement. There is no question that great advances in manual medicine have taken place in the twentieth century, but this should not blind us to the possibility that some things of value may also have been lost along the way. The last remaining osteopaths and chiropractors from Cayce's era are now passing from the scene. I think it's important to preserve some of their worthwhile legacy.

General and Specific Treatments

The Cayce readings draw a distinction between general and specific treatments, calling for "general manipulation" in some cases and "specific adjustment" or "correction" in others. In many instances, an alternation between the two types of treatment is recommended.

This demarcation between specific adjustment and general

manipulation is familiar to chiropractors, who have been taught to consider the specific adjustment the most highly evolved form of hands-on treatment. I was taught that the specific vertebral adjustment is what sets chiropractic apart from all other manual healing arts and that it is superior to all more general forms of manipulation and bodywork.

How interesting, then, to consider an alternative viewpoint which recognizes the value of the specific adjustment, but places it in a context where it is one good method among many, appropriate at some times but not at others.

What Cayce called the "adjustment," "specific adjustment," "chiropractic adjustment," or "correction," refers to what chiropractors now call a "high-velocity, low-amplitude adjustment," an "osseous adjustment," or a "traditional adjustment." This is a firm, well-controlled thrusting pressure directed at a specific vertebral level, often eliciting a popping sound as joint fixation is released.

Many changes have taken place since Cayce's time, and there are now a wide range of newer methods which contemporary chiropractors also call adjustments, but which utilize lower force or reflex techniques. Therefore, anyone attempting to apply the Cayce readings today should be aware that some translation of terms is necessary.

The general osteopathic manipulation and osteopathic massage often recommended by Cayce together comprise a kind of full-body, all-purpose, hands-on workout, which does not seek to find the source of the body's imbalance at one or two specific locations, but aims instead to release restriction, stimulate circulation, and restore overall tone through wide-ranging movements of the body's joints and muscles.

A frequent pattern in the Cayce readings was a recommendation for a few general manipulations, followed by specific adjustments at crucial spinal levels.

Stimulating and Relaxing Treatments: The Concept of Tone

Another idea often cited by Cayce is the concept of "relaxing" and "stimulating" treatments. In general, the relaxing treatments are gentler, cover a broader area, and are significantly longer in duration than the more specific, briefer, and firmer stimulating treatments.

Just as general treatments were more common in osteopathic than in chiropractic practice in Cayce's time, the relaxing methods also were more of an osteopathic specialty. There were some gentle, relaxing chiropractic methods in that era, too, among them the still-surviving Logan Basic technique, the crux of which involves a gentle, minutes-long thumb contact on the sacrotuberous ligament, a key spinal support structure located along the lower edge of the sacrum. But there is no question that, in Cayce's era, more active, forceful methods were the chiropractic profession's stock-in-trade.

Judging whether a relaxing or stimulating treatment is appropriate in a particular case requires consciously or unconsciously working with the concept of "tone." It is a common precept in many healing arts that bodily imbalances are characterized by increased or decreased tone, which can take many forms. The writings of D.D. Palmer include references to this.

Excessive tone (what we today might call "hyper" conditions) could involve symptoms like increased muscle tension, high heart rate, emotional jitters, fever, or insomnia. A state of decreased tone, by contrast, might manifest as fatigue, constipation, poor muscle tone, or excess accumulation of body fat or fluid. These examples are meant to be illustrative rather than exhaustive; a wide range of symptoms and signs can provide clues to the overall tone of the body-mind. The doctor's evaluation of tone also relies on touch and intuition, not just a specific catalog of symptoms.

While most of the examples just cited are conditions of increased or decreased overall tone, the Cayce readings also indicate that there can be areas of increased and decreased tone co-existing in the same body at the same time.

Though the evaluation of tone and the use of stimulating or relaxing treatments based on that evaluation are not specifically part of today's chiropractic college curricula, of necessity students learn this indirectly. Patients with severe osteoarthritis and rigid muscle tension, for example, are properly deemed poor candidates for forceful adjustments.

When I was in chiropractic school (and this is still true today), I was taught to use lower-force methods like pelvic blocks, Logan Basic, trigger point therapies, or reflex techniques in such cases. No one said, "This is a case of excessive tone, so therefore give a relaxing treatment," but the net effect was the same. I believe that the ability to distinguish when a relaxing treatment rather than a stimulating one is needed ranks among the most important aspects of the chiropractor's or osteopath's art.

This viewpoint, though widespread, is not universally shared by chiropractors and osteopaths. Some practitioners do not include any of the relaxing, low-force methods in their repertoires, while others use low-force techniques exclusively. My own practice has been to incorporate both approaches and to do my best to refine the art of knowing when to use each.

Drainages

The need for proper fluid balance in the body is a well-accepted physiological principle. In orthodox medicine this is often addressed only after a significant breakdown has occurred; swelling due to poor circulation, severe lymphatic blockage, and kidney failure are examples.

The approach of Cayce and the early osteopaths included methods designed to "stimulate drainages," on both a preventive and therapeutic basis. If the movement of bodily fluids is allowed to proceed unimpeded by blockage or stasis, the reasoning goes, then the toxic byproducts of metabolism will be excreted through proper channels of elimination on a regular basis, and bodily organs will not be unduly taxed by their build-up.

Techniques which overlap and supplement what Cayce called the relaxing methods were developed by the early osteopaths to aid this process. These are specific massage methods or internal organ manipulations which utilize knowledge of the body's lymphatic pathways. The body's lymphatic drainage channels all flow toward the heart; thus, drainage techniques for the upper body are geared toward moving fluids downward, and those for the lower body in general seek to move fluids upward.

Cayce frequently recommended drainage techniques for specific organs, such as the gall bladder, an organ that plays a key role in the metabolism of fats. When combined with dietary advice, such as decreasing the intake of fats and fried foods, this method offers a sensible, conservative approach designed to prevent gall bladder problems from reaching the point where more radical interventions, like surgery, are necessary.

Coordinating the Centers: Methods and Measurements

Edgar Cayce repeatedly referred to the need to "coordinate the centers." This concept, more than any other, establishes the Cayce approach among the traditional energy medicines of the world. But unlike the ancient healing arts of India and China, Cayce presents the information without the use of colorful metaphors like earth, water, fire, metal, wood, and air. To a great extent, he uses the language of modern medical science.

From Cayce's standpoint, the centers are key areas where the cerebrospinal system (the brain and spinal cord) interfaces with the sympathetic nervous system. These centers are energetic and electrical switching points. As such, malfunctions at these locations have consequences not only at the site where they occur, but much farther afield. Cayce considered coordination of the centers to be a necessary prerequisite for proper energetic balance and, therefore, health.

The most crucial of these points of interface are located at approximately the following spinal levels: C3, T4, T9, and L4 (one in the neck, two between the waist and the shoulders, and the last near the waist). Other key centers frequently noted by Cayce are the parasympathetic vagus center (originating in the upper neck, with branches into the chest and upper abdomen) and the coc-

cyx center (at the base of the spine). Again and again, Cayce emphasized the importance of coordinating these centers with one
another, either by simultaneous manual pressure at two of these
spinal levels or with very low-intensity electrical hookups.

Polarity therapy, which I learned at chiropractic school and
have used ever since, incorporates the very same concept at its
core. One of polarity's main balancing contacts for the air element and heart center, for example, involves placing one hand
on the lower back (around L4), and the other between the shoulder blades (around T4). When I first realized that this coincided
exactly with Cayce's recommendations for coordinating the centers, it was one of those wonderful "aha!" moments.

Polarity developer Dr. Randolph Stone, I realized, was trained
in both chiropractic and osteopathy in the early 1900s and, therefore, had integrated into his system many of the same basic ingre-
dients as Cayce. While Stone's and Cayce's terminology might not
be precisely the same, their approaches have a great deal in
common. Both considered balancing the centers to be crucial.

How does a practitioner determine that coordination is lacking, and how does he or she know whether a treatment has been
successful in restoring coordination? Eastern healing arts (Indian
Ayurveda and traditional Chinese medicine) use a complex and
subtle form of pulse reading to aid in this determination, but
Cayce never made reference to this method, perhaps because no
skilled practitioners of the art were available to the people who
consulted him.

More than once, Cayce mentioned a chiropractic instrument
that appears to be the Neurocalometer (NCM), a two-pronged,
heat-sensing device developed at Palmer College in the 1920s.
This, he said, could measure the coordination of the centers. The
rationale for such heat-sensing devices (there have since been
many variations) is the assumption that if the sympathetic system, which controls the nerve supply to blood vessels, is properly
balanced, it will generate skin temperatures along the spine that
are approximately equal when the right side is compared to the
left.

I was trained in the use of the NCM at chiropractic school. Like
any useful tool, if truly mastered it provides the practitioner with

a building block for the development of his or her art. Just as we can "see the world in a grain of sand," so, too, can a readout of certain physical functions provide a window into the overall workings of the human system.

While some chiropractors utilize instruments like the NCM, others seek to finely tune their own senses, evaluating temperature differences by hand. Unlike the NCM, such manual diagnosis allows comparison not only between the right and left sides, but also between higher and lower spinal levels. It also gives instant feedback, requiring no interruption of the hands-on contact between doctor and patient.

I believe the choice of methodology used to evaluate the coordination of the centers is far less important than the recognition that such coordination is necessary. Except in the elective polarity therapy course I attended, the notion of coordinating these centers was never directly addressed in my chiropractic education.

As it turns out, however, Cayce was not alone in emphasizing this concept. Irwin Korr, Ph.D., the premier osteopathic researcher of the twentieth century, considered the coordination between the cerebrospinal and sympathetic portions of the nervous system to lie at the very heart of spinal manipulative practice.

Irwin Korr, Cayce, and the Importance of the Sympathetic Nervous System

Professor Korr's landmark lecture, "The Sympathetic Nervous System as Mediator Between Somatic and Supportive Processes,"[1] draws together a broad array of research findings, arriving at conclusions remarkably aligned with the Cayce readings regarding the role of the sympathetic nervous system (SNS) and the coordination of systems and centers.

A prolific, Princeton-trained physiology researcher and writer, Dr. Korr was a genius in his ability to develop new, highly integrated interpretations of existing evidence and then to himself perform the experiments needed to fill what he perceived to be the remaining gaps in the data base. From the 1940s to the 1970s,

Korr produced an unparalleled body of neurophysiological research.

It was Korr, for example, who performed the original studies which demonstrated that nerves secrete protein substances which travel into the cellular structure of the organs they serve and that the nerve cells then receive into themselves similar substances in return. This intricate cellular give-and-take indicates a degree of communication and coordination fully consistent with the Cayce readings, one which is only now beginning to be understood by the average health care practitioner.

Korr states that the classic view of the SNS, in which its functions are largely defined by its effects on blood vessels and the smooth muscles of internal organs, is severely incomplete. He also calls for revision of the model in which the sympathetic and parasympathetic branches of the autonomic nervous system are involved in a "tug of war" and further asserts that it is inaccurate to even characterize them as equal partners. Korr is fully aware of the data from which such common conclusions are drawn, but, like Cayce, he concludes that there is far more to the picture.

Korr states that while the parasympathetic system "protects the internal environment" and "replenishes body stores depleted by SNS," the SNS itself has a far more wide-ranging role. In Korr's formulation, the sympathetic system serves as *the overall tuning mechanism for all body functions.* He places particular emphasis on SNS coordination with the muscular system, which is under cerebrospinal (voluntary) control. This squares perfectly with Cayce's fundamental assumptions about the nervous system.

The supportive research studies cited by Korr are too numerous to explain in detail here, so I'll focus on one which I found particularly interesting. In the early 1900s, the distinguished Russian physiologist Orbeli repeated a classic experiment demonstrating that stimulation of the sciatic nerve caused the gastrocnemius muscle (in the lower leg) to contract. But then he went further. He stimulated the lumbar (lower back) sympathetic nerves related to the gastrocnemius and found that this caused the muscle contraction to be greatly increased. Most remarkably, he discovered that even after the muscle reached a point of fatigue from overstimulation of the sciatic nerve, sympathetic stimulation could override the fatigue, restoring full contractile function of the muscle.

Korr notes that this crucial role of the sympathetic system, as an amplification and backup mechanism for the cerebrospinal system, has been largely ignored since Orbeli's time, presumably because it does not fit neatly into the conventional wisdom about the SNS. But the Cayce readings, with their numerous references to the need for coordinating and balancing the SNS with the cerebrospinal system, demonstrate a recognition and appreciation of the extensive scope of sympathetic function.

Cayce affirmed this to be crucial to the understanding of manipulative therapies:

> " ... the *science* of osteopathy is not merely the punching in [of] a certain segment or the cracking of the bones, but it is the keeping of a *balance*—by the touch—between the sympathetic and the cerebrospinal system! *That* is real osteopathy!"[2]

Korr discusses other studies which demonstrate that various interventions (stimulation or suppression) in the sympathetics of the neck can "impede or accelerate the rate of learning or forgetting of conditioned reflexes, and profoundly modify brain-wave patterns."[3] Moreover, in a copiously footnoted, decades-wide scan of the medical literature, Korr makes it clear that the SNS influences immune reactions, allergic responses, inflammatory processes, and the regeneration rate of injured tissues, as well as exerts a "profound influence" on cellular metabolism and on enzyme profiles in various tissues.[4]

Korr points out that most researchers on the SNS have focused on its effects related to their own particular areas of specialization—such as the digestive tract, the heart, or the lungs. What has been missing, he emphasizes, is a broad overview, in which the SNS is understood to be the primary organizing and coordinating system of the body.

The view of the SNS espoused by Korr and Cayce is still not universally accepted, despite the evidence in its favor. It requires a willingness to see the body-mind from a whole-systems perspective, in which the human being is seen as one integrated, coordinated unit, rather than a series of loosely connected parts.

Both Korr and Cayce present a paradigm in which the SNS is the structural and functional junction between mind and body, the golden central link in the chain of life. Moreover, three of the specific centers (C3, T9, and L4) most frequently mentioned by Cayce as sites for coordination between the SNS and the cerebrospinal system are prominently circled in the anatomical illustrations in Korr's paper, "The Spinal Cord as Organizer of Disease Processes: The Peripheral Autonomic Nervous System."[5] Cayce's core assumptions, it is clear, stand on solid ground.

Putting this information to good use, as part of a well-integrated manual therapeutic approach, seems to me to be a needed and worthwhile endeavor. It lies well within the scope of both chiropractic and osteopathic practice and would also be applicable by massage therapists and all others who use their hands to bring balance and healing.

TOOLS FOR SELF-HEALING

CHAPTER 11

DIET AND NUTRITION

Anyone seeking information about diet and nutrition discovers quite early that there are literally thousands of nutrition books on the market, each with a different set of rules and regulations. For the average person sincerely desiring dependable information, this presents a major dilemma: whom do you trust?

With nutrition, as with other things in life, I find it helpful to start with the assumption that many roads can lead to the desired destination. Since there are healthy people following diets that differ substantially from one another, it follows logically that no single set of guidelines must be rigidly adhered to by all people seeking good health. Fortunately, you have choices.

These choices, however, do not mean that you can eat and drink all manner of junk food in cavalier fashion, trusting that everything will turn out fine. More than likely, it won't. Some people can smoke two packs of cigarettes a day and never get lung cancer, emphysema, or asthma. Others can follow a grease-filled, vegetable-free diet, yet live to be 100 and never develop heart disease.

These people are the exceptions. For the vast majority, such courses of action have grave consequences. Unless you are blessed with a supremely strong genetic inheritance or somehow assured of a supernatural run of luck, you would be well advised to avoid these high-risk behaviors.

Health research in recent years has repeatedly turned conventional wisdom upside down. Time and again, ideas condemned as quackery by the medical establishment have appeared in learned medical journals a couple of decades later, hailed as exciting new discoveries. Perhaps the most dramatic example is the role of nutrition in cancer prevention. Scoffed at for years as a ridiculous superstition, the preventive role of a healthful diet is now heartily endorsed by the National Cancer Institute and all other major medical institutions.

Dr. Dean Ornish's research, published in the *Journal of the American Medical Association,* has scientifically proven that heart disease can be reversed through a combination of a very low-fat vegetarian diet, meditation, yoga, and participation in emotional sharing groups. No other nondrug, nonsurgical method, including the reduced-fat-plus-exercise regime which is still the standard of care in modern medicine, has ever been shown to reverse heart disease. At best, they just slow its advance.

In order to secure the funding necessary to pursue his ground-breaking study, Ornish had to edit out terms like "vegetarian" and "meditation" from his grant proposals, substituting more neutral terminology like "low fat" and "stress reduction." Fortunately, he had his priorities straight, made the required word changes, and went on to make medical history. In my opinion, Dr. Ornish's work is the single most important medical breakthrough of our generation.

We have come a long way in the past few decades. When I started studying nutrition in the late 1960s as an interested layman, the notion that ideas such as Ornish's would penetrate the bastions of the medical establishment during my lifetime seemed little more than a pipe dream. Having seen his article in the AMA's premier publication, I feel we can now set our sights even higher, aiming for a holistic, natural nutrition approach to be the recognized standard within a generation.

In certain key respects, the natural foods approach has already become the recognized standard. In the 1970s, the United States Senate Select Committee on Nutrition, chaired by Senator George McGovern, surveyed the field and then endorsed many of the long-held principles of the natural nutrition movement.

In its landmark report, this committee advised eating more whole grains, more vegetables and fruits, less salt and sugar, less meat, and less fat in general. The 1990 Dietary Guidelines of the United States Department of Agriculture, graphically represented as a pyramid in the figure on the next page, in effect codified the ideas advanced in the McGovern Committee's report. Though they do not go as far as I would like with regard to limiting meat and milk intake, they are a major step in the right direction.

In working with my patients, I find the USDA recommendations an excellent place to start. Virtually everyone can benefit from them. When this pattern truly becomes the norm, our society as a whole will be much healthier as a result. If, in addition, the entire population were to stop smoking, keep alcohol and caffeine intake to a minimum, and exercise regularly, the effects would be truly revolutionary. These simple recommendations have been repeated so often in recent years that they have become a kind of health cliché. Yet most people I see in my practice ignore at least a few of them, and some people's diets seem tailor-made for self-destruction.

Therefore, before going any further, I want to repeat as strongly as possible: *eating a low-fat, high-fiber diet centered around plant foods including whole grains, vegetables, and fruits, with highly processed junk foods kept to an absolute minimum, is the most important dietary advice I can offer you.*

If you ignore these basics and then attempt to atone by taking all sorts of pills, potions, and powders (even the good ones you find at health food stores), you are missing the boat. I am familiar with many systems of nutritional healing, some of them very detailed and demanding. I firmly believe that no esoteric set of formulas will help you as much as taking these basic, sensible, well-accepted recommendations seriously, making them part of your life on a daily basis.

Food Guide Pyramid
A Guide to Daily Food Choices

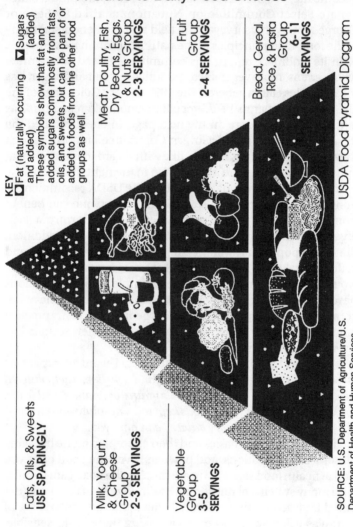

KEY
☐ Fat (naturally occurring and added) ▶ Sugars (added)

These symbols show that fat and added sugars come mostly from fats, oils, and sweets, but can be part of or added to foods from the other food groups as well.

Fats, Oils, & Sweets
USE SPARINGLY

Milk, Yogurt, & Cheese Group
2-3 SERVINGS

Meat, Poultry, Fish, Dry Beans, Eggs, & Nuts Group
2-3 SERVINGS

Vegetable Group
3-5 SERVINGS

Fruit Group
2-4 SERVINGS

Bread, Cereal, Rice, & Pasta Group
6-11 SERVINGS

USDA Food Pyramid Diagram

SOURCE: U.S. Department of Agriculture/U.S. Department of Health and Human Services

There is valuable nutritional information to be found in many sources. I have been most influenced by two:
- The low-fat, high-fiber vegetarian diet—espoused by many authors, of whom I find Dr. Dean Ornish the most knowledgeable and articulate.
- The Edgar Cayce readings—which provide the best diet I've seen for those who choose to eat meat.

These systems have broad areas of agreement, which I consider to be far more important than their disagreements.

Here are the areas of common ground:
- foods are eaten in a natural, unadulterated state
- fatty foods are kept to a minimum
- whole grains are considered far superior to processed grains and occupy an important role in the diet
- vegetables and fruits are eaten in substantial quantities
- pure water is recommended as the ideal beverage—sugary drinks and those with chemical additives are avoided
- little or no junk food is allowed—highly processed sugars, starches, and fats are eaten rarely, if at all

These basics are now widely accepted by mainstream and alternative health practitioners alike, although most conventional physicians still tend to underplay the role of a healthy diet in achieving and maintaining health.

Fortunately, you do not need a physician's prescription in order to eat a healthy diet. You can do it on your own, and I cannot overemphasize the importance of your doing so. If you choose not to act on this, you will severely handicap your chances of achieving optimal health. To the extent that a society collectively ignores this information, as is still the case in much of contemporary America, it is choosing illness over health. No amount of high-tech medical intervention can overcome this.

Charles Olson, an American poet, said we learn the simplest things last. Having in many instances reached a point of diminishing returns with regard to the role of high-tech medicine, we now have the chance to relearn these simple basic dietary principles. The time to begin is now.

Reasons for Moving Toward Vegetarianism

When people ask me whether I am a vegetarian, I answer, "Not completely." I do still have a piece of fish every now and then (several times a year on average), and someone who does this is not a true vegetarian. I believe that food cravings in some cases reflect an inner wisdom of the body-mind, and I do occasionally get a craving for fish. I don't believe that small amounts of animal food are inherently damaging, and I am open to the possibility that they may sometimes aid healing or restore strength.

However, I feel very strongly that the amount of animal flesh (mammals, birds, and fish) consumed in Western nations is drastically higher than what any human body needs, that it taxes the body severely, and is among the major contributing factors to the epidemic levels of deep-seated, chronic disease in our societies.

There is a substantial body of research indicating that the incidence of chronic, degenerative diseases like heart disease and cancer is strongly related to a high-fat, low-fiber, meat-eating diet. Even the American Dietetic Association, the national professional association of registered dietitians, which no one could call a radical fringe group, stated in 1988:

"A considerable body of scientific data suggests positive relationships between vegetarian life styles and risk reduction for several chronic degenerative diseases and conditions, such as obesity, coronary artery disease, hypertension, diabetes mellitus, colon cancer, and others . . . Vegetarians also have lower rates of osteoporosis, lung cancer, breast cancer, kidney stones, gallstones, and diverticular disease.

"Although vegetarian diets usually meet or exceed requirements for protein, they typically provide less protein than nonvegetarian diets. This lower protein intake may be beneficial, however, and may be associated with a lower risk of osteoporosis in vegetarians and improved kidney function in individuals with prior kidney damage. Further, a lower protein intake generally translates into a lower fat diet, with its inherent advantages, since foods high in protein are usually high in fat.

"It is the position of the American Dietetic Association that vegetarian diets are healthful and nutritionally adequate when appropriately planned."[1]

Some people who find out that I eat hardly any animal products ask, "But what do you do about protein?" Most of us were all trained from an early age to view protein as essential to good health. And it is essential. But the fact that a moderate amount of protein is good for us does not mean that more will be better. Where health is concerned, overdoing something can be as bad for you as underdoing it, if not worse. Western societies overdo protein, and particularly animal protein, in a big way.

John Robbins, author of *Diet for a New America* and *That All May Eat*, emphasized this point when I interviewed him:

"In this country, we derive approximately eighty percent of our protein consumption from animal products. In those parts of the world where cancers and heart disease and diabetes are much more rare, the percentage of protein consumption that comes from animal products is more like ten percent. We are consuming animal protein to a terrible excess and really damaging ourselves in the process . . . You really *can* have too much of a good thing. You can have too much sunlight, too much sleep, too much food. Certainly you can have too much protein."[2]

Because protein is a kind of "sacred cow," few people realize that it is protein excess, not deficiency, that is the greater problem for those of us in the industrialized world. In those Third World cultures where protein intake is adequate but not excessive, the diseases of Western civilization—colon cancer, breast cancer, heart disease, osteoporosis, diabetes, and kidney disease—appear quite seldom.

Dr. T. Colin Campbell of Cornell University, a former senior science advisor to the National Cancer Institute, conducted the largest study ever on the relationship between diet and health.

Campbell's research project surveyed the dietary habits of people in China and compared the results with the information available from Western countries.[3] Campbell concluded that the excess intake of animal protein and fat is the greatest cause of disease in the West. To cite merely one statistical finding from Campbell's study: a cholesterol count of 150, which in America would be considered desirably low, would be relatively high for a person in China.

In general, the Chinese diet is high in grains, beans, and soy products, vegetables and fruits. While the meat of many animals is eaten, meat forms a significantly smaller part of the typical meal than it does in the West. Furthermore, dairy products are used far more sparingly in China.

When told about the low rates of heart disease and cancer in Third World countries where people eat diets low to moderate in protein, some people respond, "That may be true, but I certainly wouldn't want to worry about dying from infectious diseases, like they do in many of those countries."

I agree, but that's not the real issue. Aside from the fact that countries with good public health and sanitation programs, like China, also have relatively low rates of infectious disease, the real question is: How can we learn from the strengths and weaknesses of both industrialized and Third World countries, creating a new path that draws on the strengths of each?

Where diet is concerned, the place to begin is by substantially limiting intake of all meats, using whole grains (brown rice, whole wheat, oats, rye, millet, and others) and legumes (beans, lentils, and soy products) in their place.

It can be done, and it's well worth the effort.

Dr. Dean Ornish's Dietary Approach

Dr. Ornish's approach draws on the wisdom of modern science and ancient tradition, and charts the way toward a future where degenerative diseases are a rarity rather than the norm.

Ornish presents two diets in his book, *Dr. Dean Ornish's Program for Reversing Heart Disease*—the Reversal Diet and the Prevention Diet. The Reversal Diet is designed for people who already have heart disease, to enable them to reverse their arterial blockages. The Prevention Diet, which is a less strict version of the Reversal Diet, is designed for people who do not have heart disease and wish to prevent it. I highly recommend reading Ornish's book, which covers the subject in detail.

You may be someone who is not particularly concerned about heart disease. If so, please remember that the same diet that prevents heart disease also prevents obesity, high blood pressure, stroke, osteoporosis, diabetes, gallstones, and cancers of the colon, breast, and prostate. These diseases are so rampant in industrialized countries that almost everyone has a close family member with one or more of these severe health problems. In most cases, these are avoidable by eating correctly.

The Reversal Diet contains ten percent fat, seventy to seventy-five percent carbohydrate, fifteen to twenty percent protein, and has five milligrams of cholesterol per day. In contrast, *the typical American diet has forty to fifty percent fat, twenty-five to thirty-five percent carbohydrate, twenty-five percent protein and has 400 to 500 milligrams of cholesterol per day.* Quite a difference!

The carbohydrate in the Reversal Diet is almost all complex carbohydrate, the kind found in whole grains, beans, vegetables, and fruits; the carbohydrate in the typical American diet is largely the simpler type found in sugar, honey, and alcohol, along with devitalized white flour products. You can eat far more of the simple carbohydrates before feeling full—and people certainly do. Complex carbohydrates are difficult for the body to convert into fat. Simple carbohydrates convert more easily. Fats in food, of course, convert most easily into body fat.

In summary, Dr. Ornish's Reversal Diet:
- is very low in fat and high in fiber
- includes no meats of any type
- excludes all oils and animal products except small amounts of nonfat milk and yogurt
- allows egg whites but not yolks (the cholesterol is all in the yolk)
- allows but does not encourage moderate alcohol consumption

- excludes caffeine, other stimulants, and MSG
- allows moderate use of salt and sugar
- is not restricted in calories

Thoughts on Edgar Cayce's Approach to Diet and Nutrition

Edgar Cayce's dietary advice, given between the early 1900s and the 1940s, was well ahead of its time in many respects. Long before such ideas were popular in America, he advocated a low-fat diet with copious amounts of fresh and lightly cooked vegetables and fruits. Whole grains, lean meats, nuts and seeds, and cultured milk products were also featured prominently.

The Cayce readings advocated treating pellagra with turnip greens as early as 1909. This was before the scientific breakthrough which identified this killer disease, a great scourge in the American South at that time, as a vitamin deficiency caused by lack of niacin (vitamin B_3).[4] Turnip greens, it is now well known, are an excellent source of niacin.

While some of the dietary recommendations in the Cayce health readings have been scientifically proven and have achieved broad acceptance in recent years, in other cases no supporting research data exists comparable in strength to that supporting the use of turnip greens for pellagra or a low-fat diet for heart disease. This does not mean Cayce's other ideas are incorrect, only that there is insufficient data currently available to scientifically determine the issue one way or the other.

With this understanding, let's explore some of Cayce's other dietary principles and suggestions.

Acid- and Alkaline-Forming Foods

Prominent in the Cayce dietary approach is his oft-repeated advice that a healthy diet should include approximately eighty percent alkaline-forming foods and twenty percent acid-forming foods.

While this may at first sound like a complicated and almost

esoteric formula to follow, in reality it is quite simple. Since the great majority of alkaline-forming foods are vegetables and fruits, it translates into a straightforward recommendation to make these a centerpiece of the diet. For many people, Cayce recommended that one meal each day consist of nothing but fresh vegetables. In essence, Cayce urged us to follow the classic advice of countless mothers and grandmothers: "Eat your fruits and vegetables!" Who could disagree?

As to the percentages, I am aware of no scientific studies that have determined what ratio of alkaline-forming to acid-forming foods is best. My advice is not to worry too much about the exact mathematical percentages, since a precise calculation is impossible without constant access to a biochemistry laboratory. The important thing is: keep eating plenty of fruits and vegetables, and don't overdo it on your consumption of acid-forming foods like meats and sweets! If you follow this advice, you'll be getting to the heart of Cayce's message, and it will do you good.

Food Combinations

Cayce also suggested that foods should be eaten in certain combinations. Appearing in various forms in many natural healing approaches, food combining is another theory which has not yet been scientifically researched.

Like the acid-alkaline recommendations, there is much anecdotal evidence supporting the idea, but the issue of food combining is so complex that devising a scientific study to prove or disprove it may be impossible. Controlling the variables would, I believe, pose problems beyond the capacities of even the most dedicated researchers.

Be that as it may, here are Cayce's proposals on food combining, which many people I know have found quite helpful in traveling the road to good health:

• Meat and starch should not be combined in the same meal. This, of course, rules out that famous mainstay of the American dinner table: meat and potatoes.

• Acidic fruits (particularly citrus) should not generally be combined with cereals or starches, other than whole wheat bread. This rules out the classic American breakfast of cereal and orange juice.

• Dairy can be eaten with vegetables and fruits, but not with starches or meats. Interestingly, this is consistent with Jewish kosher law, which declares that dairy and meat should be eaten at separate meals.

• Coffee should not be combined with cream or milk, and milk should in general be avoided altogether.

Unique Cayce Recommendations

One of the more unique Cayce recipes is the gelatin salad. He frequently advised eating raw vegetables in a gelatin mold, asserting that glandular activity is enhanced by the gelatin, thus enabling the body to more fully utilize the vitamin content of the vegetables. The readings sometimes advised combining the gelatin with specific vegetables. For example, he recommended gelatin with carrots for visual problems:

" . . . if gelatin will be taken with raw foods rather often (that is, prepare raw vegetables such as carrots often with same, but do not lose the juice from the carrots; grate them, eat them raw), we will help the vision."[5]

Here again, Cayce's insight anticipated later scientific discoveries. We now know that carrots, as an excellent source of vitamin A, are among the finest foods for the eye. It is one of nature's sweetest poetic touches that carrots and other brightly colored yellow, red, and dark green vegetables are both aesthetically pleasing to the eye and nutritionally essential for its proper functioning.

Cayce stated unequivocally that almonds could prevent cancer:

" . . . those who would eat two to three almonds each day need never fear cancer."[6]

" . . . almonds are good and if an almond is taken each day, and kept up, you'll never have accumulations of tumors . . . An almond a day is much more in accord with keeping the doctor away, especially certain types of doctors, than apples."[7]

Cayce frequently recommended the Jerusalem artichoke—a tasty, juicy tuber from the sunflower family—as a natural source of an insulin-like compound. He suggested its use for those with a tendency toward diabetes or carbohydrate intolerance or a craving for sweets. Asked by one person why she craved sweets, he said:

"This is natural with the indigestion and the lack of proper activity of the pancreas. Eat a Jerusalem artichoke once each week, about the size of a [hen's] egg . . . This will also aid in the disorder in the circulation between liver and kidneys, pancreas and kidneys, and will relieve these tensions from the desire for sweets."[8]

Cayce's readings also provide clues for future generations of nutritional researchers. In a reading for a woman with multiple sclerosis, he dropped this tantalizing hint:

" . . . keep to those things that heal within and without . . . and especially use the garden blueberry. (This is a property which someone, some day, will use in its proper place!)"[9]

How Broadly Do the Rules Apply? Principles and Particulars

One question regarding Cayce's dietary recommendations, which could equally be applied to any other set of nutritional guidelines, is the matter of how broadly they should be generalized. Do they apply world wide to all people in all cultures? If not, which aspects can best be adapted to other cultural settings?

Cayce's readings were, for the most part, given for people in the eastern and southern United States in the first half of the twentieth century. I have sometimes wondered what Cayce might have recommended for dietary healing had he been living in India, Alaska, or Peru, rather than in the American South.

To take the most obvious example, he certainly would not have recommended Cayce standbys like beef juice or gelatin to vegetarian Hindus in India. Similarly, there would have been no point in advising natives of the Peruvian Andes to eat three almonds a day, since the almond tree is unknown in their part of the world. And telling igloo-dwelling Alaskan Eskimoes to make raw salads an integral part of their diet would certainly have created practical difficulties, since few green plants grow in Arctic latitudes for much of the year.

Seen from this perspective, it seems to me it is the principles, more than the particulars, that provide the most enduring contribution of the dietary portions of the Cayce health readings. It is particularly important to keep this in mind now, as the global spread of information increases at an ever-accelerating pace. Otherwise, we risk falling into a serious conceptual error, in which we assume that because a particular diet is appropriate for people living in the temperate zone along the Atlantic Coast of the United States, it should also be followed by people in all lands and climates.

The Cayce readings recognized this:

"Do not have large quantities of any fruits, vegetables, meats, that which are not grown in or come to the area where the body is at the time it partakes of such foods. This will be found to be a good rule to be followed by all. This prepares the system to acclimate itself to any given territory."[10]

Significantly, for at least some people, Cayce placed eating locally grown foods at a higher level of priority than other dietary specifics:

" . . . use more of the products of the soil that are grown in the immediate vicinity. These are better for the body than any specific set of fruits, vegetables, grasses or whatnot."[11]

It makes sense. Through millions of years of evolution, all living beings derived their entire nutritional intake from the area where they lived. The subtle evolutionary interplay between organism and environment has taken place completely within this context. This has always been taken for granted in the greater scheme of things, until recently. We would be foolhardy to assume that a profound change in this pattern, such as the one we are now witnessing and participating in (with foods shipped to markets thousands of miles away), can be undertaken without consequences. We are participating in a grand experiment, the results of which may not turn out to be very positive.

Sometimes, deluged as we are by a flood of food facts and dietary rules, this crucial point gets lost in the shuffle. In my opinion, however, it ranks among the most important principles in the Cayce health legacy. Though among the hardest ideals for people in the modern world to achieve, eating the types of foods which are capable of growing in the area where we live and preferably foods which actually have been grown locally is a goal worthy of our aspiration. In urging us to pursue it, Edgar Cayce expressed an essential aspect of natural healing philosophy.

I have often wondered whether Cayce's recommendations would have been different if they had been given in the late twentieth century. For example, there has been a significant increase in the meat industry's use of antibiotics and hormones in the years since Cayce's death. Would Cayce still have recommended meat under these circumstances? My guess is that he would have told people to stay away from any meats that were not organically raised. People who wish to follow Cayce's health readings will have to make their own judgments on this, but I think it is important to recall that the readings were given to specific people and based on the circumstances operative at that time.

While some health principles are eternal, many aspects of agriculture have changed significantly in the past half century. Good advice on health must reflect these changes.

Food Cravings and the Wisdom of the Body

Another principle fundamental to the natural healing arts is that the body has an innate wisdom, which knows when to eat and drink, and what to eat and drink. I was taught this my first week at chiropractic school.

In listening to and analyzing all the good scientific reasons for eating more of certain foods and less of others, there is a risk of approaching food choice primarily as a left-brained intellectual exercise, one in which taste and personal desire are relegated to the background. It's important not to overdo this. Please remember to listen to your body, for it sometimes has knowledge of things that fly below the radar of the intellect.

Food cravings can sometimes be an expression of the body's inner voice. These cravings, which all people experience consciously at least some of the time, may reflect a response to legitimate biochemical and energetic needs. If you crave hot chili peppers or love to devour oranges, including the white inside the skin, this may mean that your body requires certain nutrients or energetic qualities present in these foods.

If certain foods taste heavenly to you, you may need something they contain, whether or not nutritional science has yet progressed to the point of being able to explain exactly what that something is. For example, we know that the white matter inside the skin of citrus fruits contains bioflavonoids, a part of the vitamin C complex. We know that chili peppers are an excellent source of vitamin A. Perhaps this explains why some people crave them.

But these nutrients are also found in many other foods. Why then does a particular person crave chili peppers or orange peels? Here we enter the realm of mystery and are reminded that our present understanding leaves large areas of uncertainty. In the health field, when we reach the far edges of what science can tell us, we are best advised to return to the intuitive wisdom of the body. Unfortunately, the recent and unprecedented adulteration of our food supply with chemical additives, processed sugars, and chemically altered fats, along with the steady stream of advertising propaganda for products containing them, has disrupted our natural ability to crave only what we need.

Animals in the wild, native peoples in primitive surroundings, infants unexposed to junk food, and many pregnant women retain this instinctive wisdom largely intact. The rest of us, many steps removed from the natural environment in which our ancestors evolved, retain it only in diluted form. Bearing this in mind, my advice is to be conscious of your cravings and to follow them if they are not leading you in a clearly harmful direction. There is a difference between craving a nutritious food and craving out of a habitual dependence on sugar, salt, caffeine, chocolate, or processed fats. Use your rational knowledge to supplement the raw data of your intuitive desires and you'll probably be headed in the right direction.

State of Mind When Eating

This chapter would not be complete without mentioning that there is more to nourishing the body than just choosing healthy food. Our state of mind when preparing and eating the food also influences the way it affects us. This tends to be ignored in studies of food biochemistry, but is considered by some cultures (India, for one) to be a crucial factor. These passages from the Edgar Cayce readings agree:

> " . . . *never*, [when] under strain, when very tired, very excited, very mad, should the body take foods in the system, see? And never take any food that the body finds is not agreeing with same . . . "[12]

> " . . . when worried, overtaxed . . . [food] *will not* digest . . . "[13]

I hope that reading all the serious information about nutrition in this chapter will not keep you from making your meals a time of celebration. My closing message is this: eat healthy foods, and find enjoyable ways of doing it. Eating should be a time for feeling abundance, not deprivation. If your current diet is an unhealthy one, you may go through periods of uncertainty as you readjust your diet and your tastes to a healthier life style. But I want to assure you that it is possible to craft a diet that tastes delicious and is good for you, too. It just takes a willingness to experiment.

The bibliography at the back of this book includes a list of excellent cookbooks and nutrition books to help you along the way. If you look at your local holistic bookstore, you will no doubt find other good ones as well. If your town doesn't have a good bookstore, try mail order. Don't give yourself excuses that let you put this off for some other year.

Try some of the recipes in these books. If you don't like the first ones you try, don't give up. Try some more. Keep experimenting. Enjoy! *Bon appétit!*

CHAPTER 12

EXERCISE AND YOGA

Movement is the essence of life. From the smallest proto-
zoans all the way up through the animal kingdom to the largest
whales, living beings are sustained through movement. We hu-
mans are part of this great chain of being, and we, too, thrive on
activity.

Our early human ancestors never had to plan exercise programs for themselves; their lives provided all the exercise they
needed, and then some. But with the development of civilization
and the subsequent division of labor, people whose tasks required minimal physical activity discovered that their bodies
functioned best when periods of active movement were included
in their lives on a regular basis.

The martial arts of the Orient, the yogic traditions of India, and
the classical Greek ideal of a sound mind in a sound body each
developed as unique responses to a similar calling—the natural
desire to maintain health. But they also embodied an urge to
push on to the limits of human potential. Full human develop-

ment, these traditions teach us, can best be achieved when both body and mind are given their due.

The majority of people in the modern industrialized nations are far more sedentary than typical members of agricultural or hunter-gatherer societies. This, coupled with the relatively rich diet typical among us, has created a need for more advanced knowledge of exercise physiology. We need to know what kind of exercise is best and how much of it to do. If we fail at this, the price is poorer health and shorter lives.

Exercise Physiology and Research

A great deal of modern research supports the value of regular exercise. Much of this research focuses on the health of the heart and cardiovascular system, which is understandable since heart attacks are the major cause of death in the industrialized world.

Two of the most significant studies were done by teams of researchers led by Dr. Ralph Paffenbarger of Stanford University. The first was done between 1951 and 1973 with San Francisco longshoremen. Paffenbarger showed that sedentary foremen and clerks died of coronary heart disease at twice the rate of active cargo handlers.[1] Later, Paffenbarger studied Harvard alumni and found that those who exercised regularly lived longer than those who did not. He also found that they had lower rates of heart disease, strokes, respiratory disease, and cancer.[2,3]

Numerous other studies have confirmed these findings and demonstrated a wide range of other health benefits from exercise. Michael Murphy's *The Future of the Body* provides a thorough summary of these desirable effects (this is a shortened list):[4]

- Enlarged and strengthened heart muscle
- Increased heart stroke volume
- Lowered resting heart rate
- Improved circulation
- Decreased blood pressure
- Greater bone mass
- Decreased degeneration of joints and ligaments
- Improved hormonal balance

- Strengthened immune system
- Improved resistance to cancer

Then Why Doesn't Everybody Exercise?

The data supporting an intrinsic human need for exercise is extensive and indisputable, yet many people do not exercise on a regular basis. In some cases this results from the heavy demands of work and family responsibilities. I understand this from first-hand experience; I have not always exercised as much as I needed to because I convinced myself that the time just wasn't there.

In truth, the time was there but I had decided to use it for other activities. I am certain that among the readers of this book, there are more than a few for whom this will sound uncomfortably familiar. To all of you, I want to say that it is possible to change your habits. I have done it and you can, too.

The first step in making the change is to realize that you have choices. Your future does not have to mirror the less admirable aspects of your past. Next, it helps to examine the factual information about exercise, so that any remaining doubts about the need for exercise are fully dealt with. Finally, and this is the hardest part, you must make a conscious decision to do what is required to best maintain your health over the long haul, including exercise.

You may be tempted to improve your diet first or begin other health-promoting activities like meditation, rationalizing that you can start to exercise at a later date. I want to applaud any positive step you take, but I urge you not to postpone starting an exercise program, because there really is no substitute.

You may feel that if you try just one new thing at a time, you will be more likely to hold to your commitment. This "one step at a time" philosophy works for some people, but there is also evidence that a "go for it all" approach is worth considering. In Dr. Dean Ornish's heart research, which I mentioned in the diet and nutrition chapter, it was the people who made the largest number of changes, all at once, who fared best. Dr. Sandra McLanahan, a medical physician specializing in alternative therapeutics and holistic health, who is director of stress man-

agement training at Ornish's Preventive Medicine Research Institute, describes what happened:

> "Most people think that if they just make a little change,
> they can stick to it. I think what happened to the people in
> our study is that they felt so much better [from going on the
> full program] that they stuck with it *because* they felt so
> much better."

Cutting Through Confusion

Many people don't exercise or don't do an adequate amount
of it because they aren't sure what kind of exercise is needed or
what benefits it will really bring. As is the case with nutrition,
there are hundreds of popular books on exercise, and the over-
dose of information they contain can lead to confusion. This, in
turn, can provide a ready-made excuse for inactivity. After all, if
you're not sure what to do, it's easiest not to do anything.

Confusion can also come from lack of clear purpose. That is,
why do you wish to exercise? If it's to be able to run in next year's
marathon, you will have a certain set of exercise needs, which
will differ from someone whose goal is to be able to play in a
neighborhood volleyball game without becoming too winded to
finish. If you're a weightlifter, you'll need different exercises than
if you're a swimmer.

For a great many people, myself included, the goal is just to
stay healthy rather than to engage in competitive athletics at all.
The exercise information in this chapter is presented so as to be
of value to anyone wishing to achieve and maintain health,
whether or not you see yourself as an athlete.

Aerobic Activity

It will come as a relief to many that a daily series of simple
stretching postures, along with light aerobic activity (such as
walking or bicycling) for a half-hour several times a week, provide all the essentials of a good exercise program. It is fine to do
more if you wish to attain a higher level of fitness. But if your goal

is to maintain good health, avoiding problems like arthritis and heart disease, then persistence in light exercise is the key. This bears repeating, because many people are under the impression that maintaining cardiovascular health, and therefore living longer, requires long hours of strenuous exercise.

Dean Ornish lays this misconception to rest in *Dr. Dean Ornish's Program for Reversing Heart Disease*, citing a study by Dr. Steven Blair of the Institute for Aerobics Research, which was published in the *Journal of the American Medical Association*.[5] Blair's team of researchers performed treadmill tests on over 13,000 apparently healthy people. They divided them into five groups based on fitness level and then followed them for eight years, to see if there was a relationship between physical fitness and death rates.

There was. The most sedentary group died at a much higher rate than the others. But equally interesting, Ornish notes, is the fact that the greatest difference was between the least fit group (group 1) and the second least fit group (group 2). Especially among men, there was relatively little difference between the second through fifth groups.

In other words, as Ornish concludes:

> "Walking thirty minutes a day (the activity level of group two) reduced premature death almost as much as running thirty to forty miles a week (the activity level of group five). Furthermore, in groups two through five, deaths were lower from all causes, including heart disease and cancer, when compared with the sedentary people in group one."[6]

The message is clear. Exercise is necessary, but good health does not require doing a tremendous amount. And if you wish, you can walk rather than run. This is perfectly consistent with the health readings given by Edgar Cayce, long before the word "aerobics" had been coined. Asked what exercise was best, Cayce consistently mentioned walking:

> "Walking is the best exercise, but don't take this spasmodically. Have a regular time and do it, rain or shine!"[7]

"Walking is the best exercise. Bicycling—either stationary or in the open—is well. These are the better types of
exercise. The open air activity is better."[8]

Among my favorite Cayce aphorisms is this one, which again
reminds us to get out of our chairs and walk:

" . . . after . . . breakfast to work a while . . . after lunch to
rest a while, after the evening meal to walk a mile."[9]

Running and Other Aerobic Alternatives

As a chiropractor, I agree that walking is an excellent exercise.
Among its virtues is the fact that walking, unlike many sports,
will almost never cause injury to the joints. On the other hand, I
have decidedly mixed feelings about running. I have treated patients who as a result of running have injured or aggravated
pre-existing injuries of the lower back, hips, knees, and feet.

Some people seem to thrive with running as their primary
aerobic exercise, but others do not, particularly those with a history of lower back pain. With each stride, a runner puts pressure
on the various joints of the lower half of the body. The resulting
cumulative stress can aggravate whatever imbalances are
present, resulting in increased wear and tear on the joints. Given
the choice between running and other aerobic exercise, I do not
recommend running to patients, unless they are already doing it,
have experienced no complications, and love it dearly.

There are many other ways to get your circulation moving. If you
enjoy tennis, swimming, cross-country skiing, aerobic dancing,
or any of a host of other active forms of recreation, go for it! If you
like something, you are far more likely to do it on the kind of regular basis that is required to fulfill your body's need for activity.

In recent years, a number of affordable machines have been
developed, which allow you to exercise aerobically at home. I
sometimes use a cross-country ski machine or a stationary bicycle, which allow me to exercise in the evening, the time of day I
am most likely to have a half-hour or an hour free for exercising.
Rowing and stair-walking machines are also worthwhile.

Each of these machines has its strengths and weaknesses (the bicycles and stair-machines do not exercise the upper body, for example), but all share the positive feature of providing aerobic activity. I agree with Edgar Cayce that exercise outdoors is best, and during much of the year I live up to that ideal. But it's far better to exercise indoors than not at all. Personally, I find it best not to give myself any excuses for being lazy.

Aerobic activity is a necessary part of an overall health program. But at least as important is the need for stretching, done properly and on a consistent basis.

Stretching

Have you ever watched how babies move and noticed how remarkably flexible they are? Whether touching head to toe or turning their heads in a smooth, wide arc from side to side, they put most adults to shame when it comes to flexibility. Now, think about the older people you've observed over the years. How flexible are they? It varies from person to person, of course, but in general I think we'd all agree that most seniors have but a fraction of the child's flexibility.

Based on these observations, many of us conclude, consciously or unconsciously, that there is an inevitable downhill slide that comes with the aging process. At one level, this is true. It is not fair to expect the same degree of flexibility from a seventy-five-year-old as from a five-year-old. But in a way this begs the question. The issue is not whether aging brings physical challenges, but rather how much of this is unavoidable and how soon. The truth may be far different from what we assume.

A few years ago, I attended a talk by a seventy-five-year-old man who was far more flexible than most people fifty or sixty years his junior. Rather than stand at the lectern, he sat cross-legged on a table, remarkably flexible and completely at ease as he spoke for over an hour. This was Swami Satchidananda. It has been said that it only takes one white crow to prove beyond a shadow of a doubt that not all crows are black. With regard to the question of how stiff and inflexible we must become with age, I think Swami Satchidananda is a white crow.

Perhaps we had better reexamine our assumptions. How can a septuagenarian be as flexible as the average teen-ager, if not more so? The answer is: yoga. Satchidananda brought this Indian tradition with him when he came to the United States and has trained thousands in hatha yoga methods.

Before we begin the stretching postures we all associate with yoga, it would be well to consider what Satchidananda said, when I asked him if everyone should practice yoga:

> "Yes, if you understand what is yoga . . . [It is] the tranquillity of the mind. It doesn't matter how you achieve it. You choose your own way, your own path. Maintain the tranquillity, maintain the peace. That's yoga."[10]

Yoga, then, is far more than a series of stretching postures. As you begin to practice the physical postures in this chapter, drawn primarily from Swami Satchidananda and Edgar Cayce, please begin by remembering the real purpose. Though you may be focusing your attention on the body, the body is not separate from mind and spirit. What serves one can serve the others as well. Cayce taught that "spirit is the life, mind is the builder, and the physical is the result."

Yoga and Healing

When it comes to the medical applications of yoga, Sandra McLanahan, M.D., is one of the most knowledgeable physicians in the West. I asked Dr. McLanahan how yoga differs from regular stretching exercises, and she replied:

> "Yoga is systematic in the way it changes the blood flow to various parts of the body. A study was done where 'pseudo-yoga' was compared with actual yoga postures. This was done with mentally ill patients, and the researchers found that with the actual yoga, they became much calmer and relaxed. Yoga changes brain chemistry, to increase endorphins and enkephalins, the natural opiates. Serotonin level is increased, which is associated with profound relaxation . . .

"Another difference is that in yoga, the stretching is done very slowly. Aerobics includes stretching, but it's not done slowly. *When you stretch slowly, you actually lengthen the muscle and relax the tension at the joint. When you stretch quickly, you shorten the muscle and increase the tension at the joint.* Yoga is called 'joints and glands exercise,' because it's so beneficial at increasing the blood supply to the various endocrine glands and also in releasing the stress at the joints."

Not only is it necessary to stretch slowly, but the stretches are most effective when performed in a certain order:

"You systematically increase the blood supply to different parts of the body by doing the yoga postures. They're done in a certain sequence, to move the contents of the colon along and stimulate the various glands step by step . . . You end up in a more relaxed state, because first you are doing the more intense yoga postures, the backward bends. Then you do the more relaxed postures, the forward bends. So even the progression of the postures themselves leaves you in a more relaxed state. It also lets your back relax more."

Yoga: East and West

There is a great deal of similarity between the hatha yoga of Swami Satchidananda and the exercises recommended in the Edgar Cayce readings. Some of the physical postures are identical, and the underlying concepts are perfectly in tune with one another.

Like hatha yoga, Cayce's exercise recommendations focus on the need to restore and balance the relationship between the muscular and circulatory systems of the body. One typical reading, which advised specific abdominal exercises, explained that by stimulating increased circulation, the exercises would bring "better position of the organs of the pelvis, making for better assimilations and activities throughout the bodily forces themselves."[11]

Recommending a set of exercises for one individual, Cayce said:

"We find that the exercises such as the setting-up exercise when the body first arises of a morning would be well, for this will bring strength to the lungs, vitality to the blood supply, and new life, as it were, to the muscular forces of the body. Take, then, at least five to ten minutes of exercise of the arms and limbs when the body first arises each morning."[12]

I mentioned earlier that the sympathetic nervous system controls the nerve supply to blood vessels, and that it plays a crucial coordinating role in the body. Cayce saw far-reaching sympathetic effects resulting from regular practice of a head-and-neck stretching exercise:

"For those conditions with the sympathetic system, if the body would take the head-and-neck exercise . . . it will relieve those little tensions which have been indicated . . . in head, eyes, mouth and teeth. All of these will respond to regular exercise of body and neck. It doesn't take long, but don't hurry through with it. But do regularly of morning take the time before dressing . . . we will change all of these disturbances through the mouth, head, eyes and the activities of the whole body will be improved."[13]

In numerous readings, Cayce reiterated that head-and-neck stretching exercises would prove beneficial not only for aches and pains in the head and neck, but for improving the function of various organs—particularly with regard to vision and hearing.

These exercises were often recommended in conjunction with spinal adjustments and/or massage of related areas of the spine.

Dr. McLanahan's explanation of the healing effects of yoga coincides perfectly with Cayce's recommendation of stretching exercises for "conditions with the sympathetic system." As she put it:

"Yoga also changes the neurological output, rebalancing the sympathetic in relation to the parasympathetic nervous system. Most of us are very sympathetic dominant—fight or flight. That also makes the muscles tense. It dilates the pupils, interferes with digestion, causes chronic stress to the heart, adrenals, kidneys, and everything else. Some of these yoga poses particularly increase parasympathetic nervous system activity . . . there's a lot to be said for relaxation."

The Importance of Timing

Both Cayce and Satchidananda say that it not only matters which postures you do, but when you do them. The Cayce readings consistently indicate that certain exercises are most appropriate in the early part of the day and others in the waning hours. Still others are recommended without special emphasis on when they should be done. In general, Cayce advised people to do upper body exercise in the morning and lower body in the evening.

Exercises

Warning: If any of these postures cause you pain, do not force them. Pain is a sign that you are overstepping your body's current limits.

Stretch to the point just before the pain begins, and stop there. At that point, you will be deriving benefit from the stretching, without running the risk of aggravating a muscular or vertebral problem. If your range of motion is consistently restricted, please consult a chiropractor or an osteopath who uses manipulation to ascertain the cause and, we hope, correct it.

Morning Exercises

One Cayce exercise, which I call the Big Bend, is especially recommended early in the morning, shortly after wakeup (see Figure 1). It not only stretches muscles in the legs and back, but is also an excellent deep-breathing exercise. It brings oxygen deep into the lungs and stimulates the circulation, particularly in the upper body.

For the Big Bend, rise up onto your toes, while breathing in through your nose and raising your hands high overhead. Then, as you breathe out (through the mouth or the nose), bend all the way forward so that your fingers touch your toes or come as close as you can within your range of comfort. Then breathe in again as you arise to the position in which you began, hands at your sides, standing straight and relaxed. Repeat three to ten times.

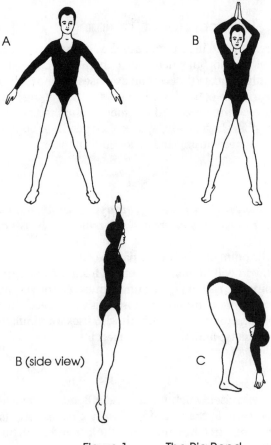

Figure 1   The Big Bend

The Big Bend is similar in some respects to the series of Indian yoga postures called Salutation to the Sun,[14] which also begins in a standing position and involves raising the hands high overhead, and then bending all the way forward, with breathing patterns that match those recommended in the Cayce readings. [Inhale on flexion (B, D, F, G, I, K) and exhale on extension (A, C, E, H, J, L).] The Salutation to the Sun (Figure 2) is more complex than the Big Bend, but there is significant overlap. As its name implies, it is also traditionally done first thing in the morning.

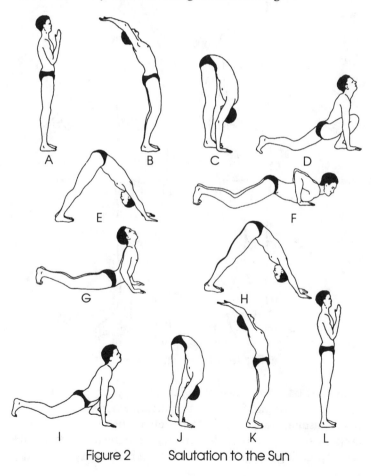

Figure 2   Salutation to the Sun

A good exercise to use just after the Big Bend and/or the Salutation to the Sun is one I call The Wheel (see Figure 3). In a standing position, feet firmly planted on the floor, rotate your body to the right and then to the left, swinging your arms as you turn first in one direction, then the other. Keep this up for at least ten turns in each direction.

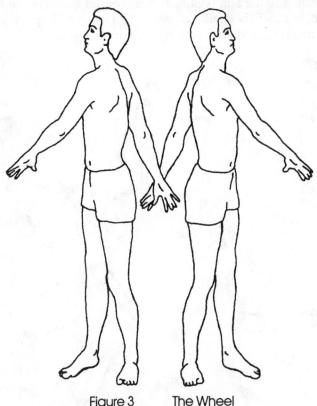

Figure 3   The Wheel

Another excellent posture to include in your morning program is the Shoulder Stand (see Figure 4), whose Indian name, Sarvangasana, translates as "a beneficial pose for the whole body." Lying on your back, lift your legs into the air, so that your feet are pointing straight up. Stabilize your back with your hands,

and press your chin forward (but not too firmly) against the upper part of your chest. Hold this posture for thirty to sixty seconds,
unless you become dizzy or uncomfortable. In this position,
blood supply is focused in the upper portion of the body. Yogic
tradition holds this to be an excellent aid in enhancing the function of the thyroid gland, which regulates the body's overall
metabolism.

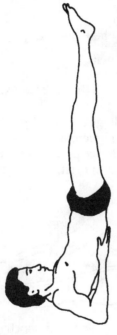

Figure 4   Shoulder Stand

Among the other time-tested yoga postures that I regularly include in my own morning series and highly recommend are
these:
    • The Upper Body Push-Up or Cobra Position (see Figure
5)—lying face down, hands below your shoulders, feet together,
elbows raised and close to the body. Slowly raise your head and
bend your neck as far back as is *comfortably* possible. After this,
raise your chest gradually, as if moving it one vertebra at a time.

Let your back do the work, not your arms as in a regular push-up. At the end, you will be looking at the ceiling (or the sky). Hold this position for a few seconds until you get used to it. Later you can do it for ten to twenty seconds.

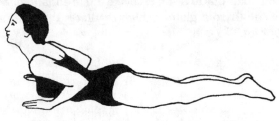

Figure 5   Upper Body Push-Up

• The Forward Bending Pose (see Figure 6)—in a sitting position, stretch your arms forward as far as you can, holding your feet, if possible, or the lower part of your legs. Hold for ten to twenty seconds, then return to sitting straight up. Repeat once.

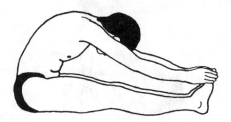

Figure 6   Forward Bending Pose

• Lying Flat on Your Back or the Corpse Position—this undramatic position with the unappealing name (Dr. Deepak Chopra renames it the "awareness pose") is an important part of a stretching session. Its inclusion in yoga is a recognition of the need for stillness to balance action. Just as silence can be a crucial element in a musical composition, lying still can play a similar role in exercise.

For this posture, you just lie on your back, legs apart, arms not touching the body, with eyes closed. Stay in that position for at least thirty to sixty seconds, longer if you wish. You may well feel that this is a waste of time, but it isn't. It functions as a sort of "reset button," allowing the body to assimilate the benefits of the other postures and enabling you to move into your day feeling calm and centered. Depending on how extensive a yoga stretching session you choose to undertake, this position may be done two or more times to punctuate the periods of greater activity.

- Head-and-Neck Stretches—One other essential part of the morning series, which can also be done at other times of day, is the head-and-neck stretching series. Time and again, Edgar Cayce recommended variations of standard head-and-neck range-of-motion exercises, the basics of which are nearly universal. I have seen books on sports medicine, chiropractic, physical therapy, yoga, and martial arts, all of which recommend essentially the same set of stretches. Recognition of the value of these exercises appears to transcend cultural and professional borders.

While there can be many individualized variations of the head-and-neck exercise, the basic model is as follows (see Figure 7).

Do not perform these exercises if they cause you to experience dizziness or nausea.)

- Bend your head straight forward (this position is called flexion), until it reaches a point of comfortable equilibrium. Let it rest there for a slow count of seven. Bring it back up to the neutral upright position. Then repeat this two more times (for a total of three), finishing with your head straight up. Breathe in and out slowly through your nose while you are stretching. Be attentive to the relaxed rhythm of your breath.
- Next, bend your head all the way back (this is known as extension), and stop when you reach a point of equilibrium, just as you did with the forward bending. As before, do this three times for a slow count of seven.
- Then, bend your head all the way to the right, bringing your ear as close as possible to your shoulder, but not so close that you feel you are straining. (This position is called

lateral flexion or side bending.) For this one, you want to bend your head to the side, without rotating it. This means that in the fully stretched position, you will still be looking straight ahead, not down or up. As with the previous stretches, do this one three times.

• Repeat the last step, except this time bend your head to the left. Three repetitions.

• Now, flex your head forward, as in the first step, and slowly roll your head around in a counterclockwise circle, three times.

• Repeat the last step, except this time circle in a clockwise direction three times.

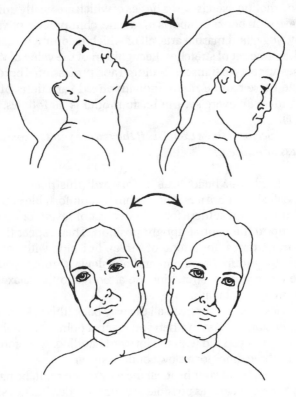

Figure 7   Head-and-Neck Stretches

Head-and-neck exercises should be included as part of your morning exercises, but are beneficial at any time of day.

• The Pelvic Rock or Cat Stretch (see Figure 8)—on your hands and knees, with hands directly below your shoulders. Curl your back up, and point your head down, forming a "C" whose ends point down. Hold for a few seconds. Then reverse the curve of the "C," with your head up and your back down. This bears a striking resemblance to the way cats often stretch, hence the traditional name of this exercise.

As you raise and lower your back and neck, be sure you are not rocking back and forth. The only movement called for is the up-and-down movement of the back and neck. The Pelvic Rock is another of the universal exercises, like the head-and-neck stretches described earlier. Not only is it used by all of the health care professions, but also in yoga and in Lamaze classes for expectant mothers.

Cayce, too, advised that "feline or cat exercise" is highly beneficial.

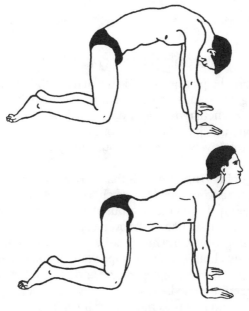

Figure 8   The Cat Stretch

• Cross-Legged Forward Bend (see Figure 9)—this is an excellent way to close your morning exercise session. Sitting in a comfortable cross-legged position, bend forward at the waist as far as you can comfortably go. If you can stretch that far, rest your forehead on the floor in front of you. Close your eyes and breathe gently. Hold this position for a minute or two, unless you begin to experience discomfort. Slowly return to an upright seated position.

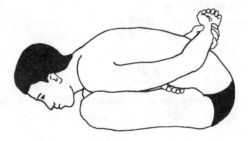

Figure 9   Cross-Legged Forward Bend

Stretching During the Day

Aside from the planned exercises you do in the morning and the evening, there may be times during the day when you feel tension in a particular muscle and wish to do something to relax it. This happens to just about everyone at least occasionally, and most of us intuitively try to figure out what position will relieve the stress.

The key point to remember is that muscles, which have been contracted for a while, need to stretch. This stretching should be done frequently during the day, but all of us forget sometimes. Therefore, if you have been bent over a desk in rigorous concentration reading a book and have hardly stirred from that position for the past two hours, it is very important for you to stretch the muscles which have been contracted and contract the muscles that have been stretched.

The way to do this is to move your body into a position approximately equal and opposite to the one you have been in. So, if you have been bent over the desk with your body flexed forward, the appropriate equal and opposite exercise would be for you to stretch back, extending the spine, contracting the muscles along the spine, and at the same time stretching the muscles of the abdomen and chest.

The opposite need arises if you have been in a position of extension (bending backward) for a longer than normal period of time. This is a less common problem, but not unknown. Patients of mine who are divers, mechanics, and plumbers, for instance, sometimes have to keep their backs or necks in extension for long periods.

To compensate for this, there is a need to flex the trunk or neck, bending forward. There are a number of good ways to do this. If the social circumstances are appropriate, you can lie on the floor and roll your body into a ball, in the fetal position. If that will raise too many eyebrows, you have the option of sitting in a chair (or on the floor) and bending forward for fifteen to thirty seconds, stretching out those tense back muscles. Ideally, each muscle group in the body should be contracted and stretched numerous times on a typical day. Figure out (or ask your chiropractor) which muscles you need to stretch during the day, and then be consistent about stretching them. This regimen will lead to a body in good balance.

Stretches for the Evening

Lower body exercise late in the evening helps you relax and prepare for sleep. Cayce consistently advised this as a way of staying in sync with what are essentially rhythmic circulatory tides in the body.

He put it this way:

> "The natural tendency . . . of [the] system is upper circulation . . . during the day, and . . . trunk circulation during the evening."[15]

If you are considering beginning an evening exercise program, but are hesitant to do so because you're just too tired at that time of day, consider the following advice, given by Edgar Cayce to someone who asked the very same question:

> "The best way to acquire the correct amount of pep is to take the exercise!"[16]

To begin a modest program of evening exercise, I suggest the following. (These exercises shouldn't take more than five minutes or so and they do the job well.)

• The Pelvic Roll—with your feet against a wall, and your hands and body in a "push-up" position, rotate your pelvis from side to side (see Figure 10). Begin with several of these rotations, and then increase gradually from there, up to forty repetitions.

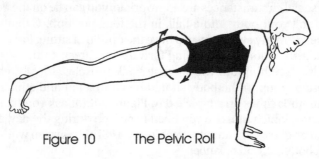

Figure 10   The Pelvic Roll

• Knee-Chest Stretch (see Figure 11)—lying on your back, bring one bent knee up toward your chest and hold it there for a few seconds. Then let it back down, stretching it out fully. Repeat with the other leg, and then with both legs at the same time. Repeat these three maneuvers four times when you are beginning. This is probably the most commonly recommended exercise for lower back pain.

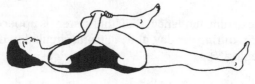

Figure 11   Knee-Chest Position

- Knee-Over Twist (see Figure 12)—lying on your back with both legs stretched out fully, bring your left knee up at a right angle (so that your thigh is perpendicular to the floor). Keeping your shoulders flat on the floor, twist your waist, bringing the left knee as far over as you can toward the floor on your right side. Hold for a few seconds, and then bring your knee back up and return to the starting position. Repeat with the other leg. Go through this exercise three times with each leg.

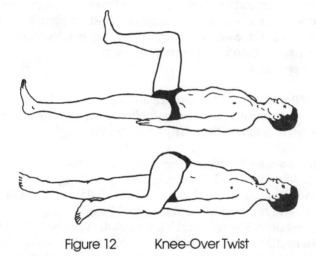

Figure 12   Knee-Over Twist

Dr. Harold Reilly, who worked with the Cayce readings as a physical therapist for forty-five years, says these "horizontal exercises have a tendency to normalize the circulation and take the strain off the arterial capillaries and veins of the lower extremities [legs]."[17] Reilly provides two dozen "P.M. Horizontals" in *The Edgar Cayce Handbook for Health*, an excellent resource book.

The Importance of Breath

One of my earliest memories is of the time when I first noticed my breathing. I was no more than two or three years old, and I recall becoming totally fascinated by the way my abdomen went in and out and by the fact that I could control its movement by whether I let air in and out through my mouth or nose. Until that day, my breathing had been completely unconscious.

Breathing is one bodily function which we can either control voluntarily or put on "automatic pilot." For the purpose of getting enough oxygen to stay alive, no effort is usually required. But to attain optimal health, breathing exercises are worth learning.

Both the Cayce readings and yoga traditions place a strong emphasis on the use of these conscious breathing techniques. Since our respiration during sleep is slower and more shallow than while awake, these exercises are most frequently recommended for the early morning. They bring needed additional oxygen to the blood, helping to wake us up.

Cayce said:

"Breath is the life-blood cleansing of the body . . . For, there are the needs for the combination of the gases as inhaled to act upon the purifying of the system."[18]

There are several types of breathing techniques:
• Alternate Nostril Breathing: These techniques utilize alternating patterns of inhalation and exhalation through the mouth and the right and left nostrils. The breathing should be slow and deep. The right and left nostrils are understood to have different effects on body energetics. Indian tradition calls breathing through the left nostril the Moon Breath and breathing through the right nostril the Sun Breath. Cayce said, "The left nostril is the spiritual, or the easing; the right nostril is the strength. So keep 'em balanced!"[19]

Here are a few of the many patterns of alternative nostril breathing:
(1) Close right nostril with thumb, then fully exhale slowly through the left nostril. Slowly inhale through the left. Then close left nostril with fourth and fifth fingers and exhale through the right. Then inhale through the right. Continue to alternate sides.
(2) Breathe in through the left nostril, and then out through the mouth. Then in through the right, and out

through the mouth. Continue to alternate.

(3) Breathe in through the left nostril, and out through the left nostril. Repeat three times. Then breathe in through the right and out through the left. Repeat three times.

• Slow, Deep Breathing: Most yogic breathing exercises utilize controlled deep "abdominal" breathing. As you inhale, first fill the lower portion of the lungs. As you do so, your abdomen will visibly expand. As the lower part of the lung fields is filled, continue to inhale, filling the chest as well. To inhale slowly and steadily, it is best to partially close the glottis (in the back of your throat), so that the air is being pulled into a now-narrowed upper end of your breathing passage. (This is best learned in person from a yoga teacher.)

• Forceful Breathing Exercises: With these methods, it is important to stop if you become dizzy. These exercises can serve as an excellent "wake-up call" at any time of day. It is good to include one in the morning exercise series.

(1) In a squatting position, feet flat on the floor (leaning your back against a wall if you need to), bring your elbows to the inside of your knees, inhaling deeply through the nose as you use your elbows to slowly push your knees apart from each other. Then exhale fiercely through the mouth, letting out the sound "Ha!" as you exhale. Repeat no more than five times. (See Figure 13.)

(2) Sitting in a comfortable cross-legged or seated position, breathe in forcefully through the nose, and then quickly and forcefully pull in your diaphragm and expel the air through the nose. Repeat several times. When you finish, inhale slowly and deeply. You can increase the number of repetitions after you get used to this technique, which in yoga is called "Skull Shining."

(3) Follow the same directions as #2, except exhale more forcefully than you inhale. After one inhalation and exhalation, inhale slowly and deeply, filling the lungs. Hold your breath as long as is comfortable and bend your head forward so that your chin comes as close as possible to your

chest. Exhale as you raise your head back up. Repeat a few times. This exercise is called "Bellows Breathing."

(4) In a standing position, hold your hands in front of your solar plexus area. Push them forward abruptly, as you exhale forcefully making the sound "Shhhi!"

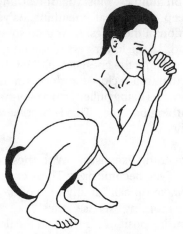

Figure 13   Squatting Position

In developing your own personal exercise program, it is helpful to learn traditional techniques and postures, but always remember that each person is unique and that your specific needs may require some variation from the specifics given in this or any other book. If possible, consult a yoga teacher or knowledgeable health professional with questions about how this information applies to you. If you have a history of neck or back problems, consulting a chiropractor or osteopath prior to beginning an exercise program is highly recommended.

CHAPTER 13

MEDITATION
AND RELAXATION

For thousands of years, religions the world over have extolled
the benefits of meditation and quiet contemplation. In Islam and
Catholicism, Judaism and Buddhism, Hinduism and Taoism, and
in religious practice from the Americas to Africa to Asia, the value
of sitting quietly, using various techniques to cultivate stillness
or focused attention of the mind, has been well recognized.

The goals of religious meditation extend far beyond its potential physical health benefits and also extend beyond the scope of
this book. Higher human function of body, mind, and spirit is
explored in sacred literature throughout the world. An excellent
summary of ancient and contemporary information on the subject can be found in Michael Murphy's landmark book, *The
Future of the Body: Explorations into the Further Evolution of Human Nature.*

In the closing years of the twentieth century, the intimate connection between body and mind is widely acknowledged. Once
the domain of speculation by mystics and philosophers, this

realm has in recent decades been visited and revisited by scientists, who have produced an impressive array of documentation. Most of this research appeared after 1970, and there currently exists a state of informational jet lag, in which the available documentation has not yet fully percolated through the scientific community. Thus, meditation remains a tool drastically underutilized within the medical fields.

The data pool is now so substantial that it can be stated, without fear of contradiction, that meditation and related relaxation techniques have been scientifically shown to be highly beneficial to health. Over a thousand research studies, most of them published in well-respected scientific journals, attest to a wide range of measurable improvements in human function as a result of meditative practices.

Herbert Benson, M.D., and the Relaxation Response

Herbert Benson's research at Harvard in the early 1970s led the way. Benson's impeccable credentials and university affiliation, along with the world-class quality of his work, led to publication of breakthrough articles on meditation in the *Scientific American* and the *American Journal of Physiology.* His book, *The Relaxation Response*, topped the best-seller lists in the mid-1970s and is still widely read.

In *The Relaxation Response*, Benson concluded, based on his research, that meditation acted as an antidote to stress. The body's physical response under stress is well known; when a real or imagined threat is present, the human nervous system activates the fight-or-flight mechanism. The activity of the sympathetic portion of the nervous system increases, causing an increased heart beat, increased respiratory rate, elevation of blood pressure, and increase in oxygen consumption.

This fight-or-flight response has a purpose. If you need to run quickly to escape an attack by a wild animal or need increased strength to battle an invader, you will be better equipped to do so if the fight-or-flight mechanism is turned up to maximum intensity. But this mechanism functions best when used occasionally, for brief periods only. If activated repeatedly, the effects are harmful and potentially disastrous. It is not uncommon for people in modern societies to maintain high stress levels most of the time. The current epidemic of hypertension and heart disease in the Western world is in part a direct result.

The effects of meditation, Benson demonstrated, are essentially the opposite of the fight-or-flight response. Benson's research showed that meditation:

- Decreases the heart rate
- Decreases the respiratory rate
- Decreases blood pressure in people who have normal or mildly elevated blood pressure
- Decreases oxygen consumption

These basic findings have been replicated by so many subsequent studies that they are not in dispute. They also established once and for all that meditation is physiologically distinct from sleep. In sleep, oxygen consumption drops about eight percent below the waking rate, and this decrease occurs slowly over a period of five or six hours. In meditation, it drops ten to twenty percent in minutes. Moreover, alpha waves, which indicate a state of relaxed alertness, are abundant during meditation and rarely noted in the sleep state.[1]

Meditation's Effects on Muscle Tension and Pain

Numerous studies have shown a decrease in muscle tension during meditation. As Michael Murphy points out, this "contributes to the body's lowered need for energy, the slowing of respiration, and the lowering of stress-related hormones in the blood." In some studies, the decrease in muscle tension as a result of meditation even exceeded the impressive effects of biofeedback training. One interesting study measured the electrical patterns in muscles and demonstrated that the lotus position (seated with legs fully crossed), a traditional posture for meditation, is the only position in which the body's muscles are as relaxed as they are when lying down.[2]

Meditation has also been shown to aid in the alleviation of

pain. Extensive studies on chronic pain patients have been conducted by John Kabat-Zinn, Ph.D., the founder and director of the Stress Reduction Clinic at the University of Massachusetts Medical Center and associate professor of medicine in the Division of Preventative and Behavioral Medicine at the University of Massachusetts Medical School. Kabat-Zinn and his program were featured on the American public television (PBS) series *Healing and the Mind*, with Bill Moyers.

Dr. Kabat-Zinn's studies have demonstrated decreases in many kinds of pain in people who had been unresponsive to standard medical treatment. A large majority of the patients in Kabat-Zinn's studies who were taught to meditate improved, while control groups of similar patients showed no significant improvement. Various related studies have shown decreases in pain from muscle tension, headaches, dysmenorrhea, and other conditions.[3]

Changes in Brain Waves and Enhanced Perception

It should come as no surprise that among the well-documented effects of meditation is the alteration of brain-wave patterns. Dozens of studies have shown an increase in alpha rhythms, which are correlated with a state of relaxed alertness. In addition, numerous studies have shown enhanced synchronization of alpha rhythms among four regions of the brain—right, left, front, and back. This may be an indication of increased coherence of brain-wave activity.[4]

Some researchers have demonstrated positive effects of meditation on mind-body coordination, exploring this area by measuring such parameters as visual sensitivity to light flashes,[5] response to auditory stimuli,[6] and the ability to remember and discriminate musical tones.[7] There are also indications that during meditation the function of the right hemisphere of the brain (generally correlated with creativity and imagination) is enhanced, while that of the left hemisphere (generally correlated with linear, intellectual thought) is inhibited.[8]

Despite the encouraging trend of increased research attention to the subject in recent years, scientific evaluation of meditation is still in its early stages. While certain benefits have been proven, much remains untested. Furthermore, the technology may not yet exist to validate many of the most profound effects of meditation. It is likely that research in the coming decades will take us far beyond our current knowledge, just as today's level of understanding far exceeds that which existed prior to 1970.

Meditation Methods

Now that the value of meditation has been established, one might reasonably ask: What exactly is meditation, and how do I meditate? Ironically, these questions are not easy to answer, because there are so many different approaches.

Most widely used meditation methods evolved as part of religious traditions and, as such, each of them may be controversial for people who do not identify with the tradition in which the particular method developed. Since this is a book on health rather than religion, I want to tread lightly when discussing religious meditation. I personally have found value in meditative techniques of religious origin, whether it has been the Vedic roots of Transcendental Meditation (TM), the Judeo-Christian orientation of Edgar Cayce's method, or the Buddhist origin of various Tibetan, Chinese, or Japanese practices.

I have personally practiced several of these techniques and feel that I have benefited from each. But out of respect for all who have qualms about mixing their health care with religion, when I speak to patients about meditation I always encourage use of a method consistent with *their own beliefs*. I usually say something like, "I'm not selling a particular brand." I also emphasize to my patients, and wish to reiterate here, that the physical health benefits of meditation can be attained through the practice of any of the methods in this chapter and through other methods as well.

The Relaxation Response

Aside from generating ground-breaking research, it may be that Dr. Herbert Benson's most lasting contribution is the development and popularization of a meditative technique with no religious overlay. This approach allows those who are not religious or whose beliefs may appear to conflict with the teachings connected to a particular meditation system to nonetheless participate fully in this worthwhile, health-giving activity.

According to Benson, the relaxation response technique produces the same physiological changes as does Transcendental Meditation, the method which has been most fully researched in scientific settings.

Here are Benson's directions for evoking the relaxation response:

(1) Sit quietly in a comfortable position.

(2) Close your eyes.

(3) Deeply relax all your muscles, beginning at your feet and progressing up to your face. Keep them relaxed.

(4) Breathe through your nose. Become aware of your breathing. As you breathe out, say the word "ONE" silently to yourself. For example, breathe IN. . . OUT, "ONE"; IN. . . OUT, "ONE"; etc. Breathe easily and naturally.

(5) Continue for ten to twenty minutes. You may open your eyes to check the time, but do not use an alarm. When you finish, sit quietly for several minutes, at first with your eyes closed and later with your eyes opened. Do not stand up for a few minutes.

(6) Do not worry about whether you are successful in achieving a deep level of relaxation. Maintain a passive attitude and permit relaxation to occur at its own pace. When distracting thoughts occur, try to ignore them by not dwelling upon them and return to repeating "ONE." With practice, the response should come with little effort. Practice the technique once or twice daily, but not within two hours after any meal, since the digestive processes seem to interfere with the elicitation of the relaxation response.[9]

Transcendental Meditation
and the Use of Mantras

TM was brought to the Western world in the mid-twentieth century by Maharishi Mahesh Yogi, an Indian spiritual teacher. The Maharishi's method has been taught to hundreds of thousands of people and is widely credited with being the first form of Eastern meditation to be practiced on a mass scale in the West.

Herbert Benson's original research subjects were TM practitioners (they were the ones who approached him with the idea of doing research on meditation), and it is TM that Benson used as the basis for formulating his relaxation response method. The relaxation response incorporates many of the principles of TM, but with the Indian tradition removed. TM organizations assert that something significant is lost when the traditional methods are not followed in full.

I cannot provide a step-by-step series of instructions for TM as I did for the relaxation response, because those who receive instruction in TM agree not to reveal the details of what they have learned. I feel it is appropriate to share certain general principles of the TM teachings, however, since they may well be applicable elsewhere. TM is presented as a method that involves neither concentration nor contemplation. That is, unlike some meditative practices, you do not attempt one-pointed focus on an idea or a visual image nor do you pursue trains of thought, however interesting, worthwhile, or inspired they may seem.

Instead, you use a mantra (a seed-syllable or primordial sound) given to you by a TM teacher. The sounds used for mantras, which are derived from Sanskrit, do not have a verbal meaning and thus are not intended to engage the cognitive mind. The mantra is a sound you say silently to yourself, which functions something like the ringing of a bell. Just as Benson used the word "ONE" in the sample directions given for the relaxation response, TM practitioners use their mantras to help still the mind when distracting thoughts intrude.

The internal chatter created by these thoughts is a normal occurrence. (What shall I wear this morning? How will I ever solve that problem at work?) But meditation time is not for working on problem solving. When such a thought arises, you should acknowledge it, and then let it pass, silently repeating the mantra to yourself.

Eknath Easwaran, an Indian-born meditation teacher, philosopher, and author, speaks of the purpose of the mantra in his book, *Meditation*. He says, "Our aim, remember, is to drive the mantra to the deepest levels of consciousness, where it operates not as words but as healing power."[10]

For those who do not practice TM, some possible mantras from various traditions are:

- Peace
- Love
- Om Mani Padme Hum
- Om Nima Shivaya
- So Hum
- Hari Om
- Tat Twam Asi
- Thank You
- Be Still, and Know That I Am God
- The Lord Is My Shepherd
- Thy Will Be Done

It is common for beginners at meditation (of all types) to experience a great deal of mental chatter and clutter. If this happens to you, it does not mean that you are doing anything wrong. Just notice each thought as it comes, and then let it pass on by, using the mantra, as it were, to break the spell. As a rule, people who are patient enough to continue the practice of meditation for months or years notice gradual changes in the ratio between silence and internal chatter. Step by step, there is more silence and less chatter. Even experienced meditators, however, are likely to have periodic increases in the amount of internal chatter, especially in times of stress.

Deepak Chopra on
Meditation and Health

Deepak Chopra, M.D., is a physician and author who practices TM. Trained as an endocrinologist, he now practices traditional Indian Ayurvedic medicine (which emphasizes the use of herbs and meditation) in Massachusetts and has authored several best-selling, highly influential books on holism, the best known of which is *Quantum Healing*. Dr. Chopra also serves on a review panel for the National Institutes of Health Office of Alternative Medicine.

In his book, *Unconditional Life: Discovering the Power to Fulfill Your Dreams,* he provides a set of questions with which to evaluate meditative practices:

> "There are any number of important issues to consider when evaluating a form of meditation—above all: Did my mind actually find the silence I was seeking? Was I psychologically comfortable during and after meditation? Did my old self begin to change as a result of having meditated? Is there more truth in my self?"[11]

For Dr. Chopra, TM provided what he sought. Similarly, I know people who have practiced TM for years, enjoy it greatly, and find it to be supportive of their physical well-being and personal growth.

I interviewed Dr. Chopra and asked how he views the relationship between meditation and healing. His answer draws on some of the concepts explored in depth in *Quantum Healing:*

> "Our bodies ultimately are fields of information, intelligence, and energy. Quantum healing involves a shift in the fields of energy information, so as to bring about a correction in an idea that has gone wrong. So quantum healing involves healing one mode of consciousness, mind, to bring about changes in another mode of consciousness, body.
>
> "Meditation is a very important aspect of all the ap-

proaches that one can use in quantum healing, because it allows you to experience your own source. When you experience your own source, you realize that you are not the patterns and eddies of desire and memory that flow and swirl in your consciousness. Although these patterns of desire and memory are the field of your manifestation, you are in fact not these swirling fluctuations of thought.

"You are the thinker behind the thought, the observer behind the observation, the flow of attention, the flow of awareness, the unbounded ocean of consciousness. When you have that on the experiential level, you spontaneously realize that you have choices and that you can exercise these choices—not through some sheer will power, but spontaneously."[12]

I asked Chopra whether he felt that TM was superior to other forms of meditation, and his answer reflected a broad-minded respect for other approaches:

"I feel that all forms of traditional meditation which are time-tested are worthwhile. My experience is with TM, therefore I am best qualified to speak about TM . . . My experience is that it is effortless, easy, spontaneous. It allows the mind to simply transcend to its source. This does not mean I think Zen is not a good form of meditation or that Vipassana is not. They are all authentic forms of meditation. That is why they have survived over thousands of years."[13]

The quest for profound inner silence and stillness is the essence of meditation. Chopra illumines this beautifully in the following passage from *Unconditional Life*, as he converses with a patient who has had anxiety attacks since childhood. The man is concerned that he never actually experiences periods of silence in meditation.

" 'But intellectually,' I [Chopra] said, 'you realize that the mind can be silent?'

" 'Not mine,' he said.

" 'Why not?'

" 'It's too quick.'

" 'But even a quick mind has gaps between thoughts,' I pointed out. 'Each gap is like a tiny window onto silence, and through that window one actually contacts the source of the mind. As we're talking here now, there are gaps between our words, aren't there? When you meditate, you take a vertical dive into that gap.'

" 'Sure, I can see that,' he rejoined, 'but I don't think I experience it in meditation.' I asked him what he did experience. He said, 'The only thing that makes meditation different from just sitting in a chair is that when I open my eyes after twenty minutes, I often feel that only two or three minutes have passed—I am intrigued by that.'

"I said, 'But you see, this is the very best clue that you have gone beyond thought. When you don't have thoughts, there is silence. Silence does not occupy time, and in order to contact the Self, one has to go into the field of the timeless. Your mind might not be able to register this experience at first, because it is so accustomed to thinking. You may feel that time has simply flown by, or that it was lost somewhere. But the "lost" time was actually spent immersed in the Self.' "[14]

Meditation as Taught by Edgar Cayce

The Cayce method was my first introduction to meditation and is one to which I have returned in recent years. I am particularly attracted to its underlying intention—the integration of body, mind, and spirit. The goal of meditation, say the Cayce readings, goes beyond attunement within the individual; it includes service to humankind and a heightened relationship to God or the Creative Forces.

"What *is* meditation? . . . it is the attuning of the mental body and the physical body to its spiritual source . . . it is the attuning of . . . physical and mental attributes seeking to know the relationships to the Maker. *That* is true meditation."[15]

Cayce said that we must learn to meditate, just as we once learned to walk. It is very important not to mistake beginnings for failures. We each must begin at the beginning and should understand that we may falter in some of our early steps. The place to start, Cayce asserted, is not with technique but with an examination of our purpose. Find your ideal, he urged, so that your practice of meditation will be grounded in a positive purpose. This ideal might be "love," "compassion," "serving others," or any of a host of other worthwhile guiding principles. What matters most is that it truly be an ideal that embodies service and that it be something you have a sincere commitment to live up to.

In her book, *Healing Through Meditation and Prayer*, Meredith Puryear offers a clear and concise introduction to Edgar Cayce's approach to meditation. Before laying out a specific set of directions, Puryear asks us to remember why we are meditating and offers suggestions on how to enhance the effects of meditation:

"When we ask how to meditate, the real question we are asking is: How do we learn to commune with God? The answer lies not in some technique, though every activity will have some form to it, but with the desire of the heart to know our oneness with Him. To awaken this desire we must feed our soul and mind a more spiritual diet. We must begin to take time to listen to beautiful, uplifting music, to read inspirational poetry and prose and the great scriptures of the ages: the Bible, the Koran, the Talmud, the Bhagavad-Gita.

"Even five minutes a day with some uplifting word will change the direction of our lives. We must also make some real choices about the kind of reading, TV, and movie diet we choose . . . These choices involve voluntary use of time, energy, and money; they also entail involuntary glandular involvement, because the glandular centers and secretions play a part in every activity of our lives. With every activity in which we engage, we are building toward something either constructive or destructive. The choices themselves may at first be a matter of discipline; but as we continue to do with persistence what we know to do, we will find it becoming easier and easier, because the process of meditation or communion changes our desires, and we begin to want different things and activities than we had heretofore."[16]

The following set of directions for meditation is adapted from Puryear's book, which in turn is based on the Cayce readings[17]:

(1) Set the ideal

(2) Set a time—be regular, persistent, and patient

(3) Prepare—physically, mentally, spiritually

Physical Preparation:

- Posture: spine straight (sitting on chair with feet on floor, lying on back, or sitting cross-legged)
- Head-and-neck exercise (for these exercises, see p. 179
- Breathing exercise (for a few alternative preparatory breathing exercises, see "Alternate Nostril Breathing" p. 186)

(4) Invite protection—Surround yourself with the consciousness of the presence of the Christ Spirit (alternatives might include surrounding yourself with the love of God, a pure white light, or any other healing and uplifting image or thought)

(5) Use an affirmation—Cayce recommended beginning with the Lord's Prayer. This may be followed by a specific affirmation, such as "Make me an instrument of Thy peace." (You may, as always, substitute any phrase which has deep meaning for you.)

(6) Silence!

Return to the affirmation (or a shortened version of it) as distracting thoughts arise. Continue for ten to thirty minutes or whatever period of time feels intuitively appropriate to you.

(7) Pray for others

What is called the "affirmation" in these directions is the structural equivalent of the mantra in TM and the word "ONE" in Dr. Benson's relaxation response method. It is the meditator's all-purpose tool, the one used for prying ourselves out of all the dead-end nooks and crannies the mind invents to distract us from the depths of silence and the heights of revelation.

Edgar Cayce said that "Meditation is listening to the Divine within."[18]

May we all become good listeners.

CHAPTER 14

VISUALIZATION, AFFIRMATIONS, AND PRAYER

As Bernie Siegel, M.D., notes in *Love, Medicine, and Miracles*, medical statistics can lead both doctors and patients to assume the worst, at a time when hope is essential. Though the statistical odds may be ninety-nine to one against recovery from a particular severe illness, there is no way of knowing in advance which one of the next 100 people will be the survivor. Or which two, or three, or more.

Similarly, when a doctor gives a prognosis (predicted outcome) on any case of any kind, he or she is making what amounts to an educated guess. The truth is that no physician ever knows the course of a patient's healing process in advance. It is the doctor's responsibility to share the information he or she has, based on scientific research as well as personal experience. But all patients should remember that each case stands on its own, and its outcome is *not* dependent on something that happened elsewhere to other people, no matter how large the statistical sample and no matter how compelling the research documentation.

This applies whether we are talking about a surgeon forecasting the life expectancy of a cancer patient or a chiropractor predicting the length of time a patient will need to recover from severe lower back pain. Patients should, if at all humanly possible, never assume that they are limited to the time frame in a doctor's prognosis. Otherwise, the prognosis becomes a strait jacket at best, a death sentence at worst.

But just as negative thinking can limit us, positive thinking can mobilize our healing powers. When this occurs, the effect goes beyond the facilitation of physical healing; an enhanced sense of personal purpose and meaning can emerge as a by-product.

One of the pioneer works documenting the power of the mind in healing is *Getting Well Again*, a 1978 book by O. Carl Simonton, M.D., Stephanie Matthews-Simonton, and James Creighton. Dr. Simonton, a radiation oncologist, got his first inkling of the power of the mind in healing early in his career when, as a physician at Travis Air Force Base in California, he ran a research study of 152 cancer patients and found that *"a positive attitude toward treatment was a better predictor of response to treatment than was the severity of the disease."*[1]

This led Simonton in a new direction, in which he combined visualization exercises and counseling with the standard radiation therapy, and found that many of his cancer patients achieved outcomes far better than expected.

After learning a progressive relaxation exercise (see Appendix), in which they mentally relaxed their bodies step by step, the patients visualized their cancers being overwhelmed by "tiny bullets of energy." Then they pictured their weakened and dying cancer cells being flushed out through their livers and kidneys by their own white blood cells. Simonton's stunning results generated great controversy within the medical profession, since they confounded the then-current conventional wisdom that cancer was something that "happens to people," something over which patients can exert little or no personal control.

Simonton described his initial results as follows:

"In the last four years, we have treated 159 patients with a diagnosis of medically incurable malignancy. Sixty-three of the patients are alive, with an average survival time of 24.4 months since the diagnosis. Life expectancy for this group, based on national norms, is 12 months . . . With the patients in our study who have died, their average survival time was 20.3 months. In other words, the patients in our study who are alive have lived, on the average, two times longer than patients who received medical treatment alone. Even those patients in the study who have died still lived one-and-one-half times longer than the control group."

After four years, the status of the patients still living was as follows:

	Number of Patients	Percent
No evidence of disease	14	22.2%
Tumor regressing	12	19.1%
Disease stable	17	27.1%
New tumor growth	20	31.8%

Simonton reminds us to "keep in mind that 100 percent of these patients were considered medically incurable."[2]

These findings, which were published in the *Medical Journal of Australia*, stood the test of time. As detailed in Simonton's 1992 book, *The Healing Journey*, follow-up reports were obtained on ninety-eight percent of the patients in the original study, and their survival times were twice those achieved at the world's leading cancer centers.

Skeptics have argued that Simonton, a man whose reputation has been built on using the power of the mind to facilitate physical healing in cancer patients, may not qualify as a credible and unbiased observer. And Simonton himself admits that due to limited funds, his initial study lacked "the randomization, and a matched control population, necessary for maximum scientific credibility."[3]

At the time of Simonton's initial studies, no scientifically airtight research existed to demonstrate the powerful effect of the mind in surviving cancer. There is now such a study. In 1989 a controlled, randomized study on women with advanced breast cancer was published by researchers at Stanford and the University of California at Berkeley, led by Dr. David Spiegel of Stanford. They reported that rates of survival among those who received counseling were twice the national average, and their statistics matched Simonton's percentages almost exactly. *This study was conducted by researchers who did not expect that counseling would have any effect on cancer survival rates.*[4]

While Spiegel's research utilized counseling rather than visualization, the results were comparable, and the central point had been made: our thoughts and emotions are intimately related to our health status.

In gradually increasing numbers, physicians and other health care providers have incorporated healing imagery into their work. Psychiatrist Gerald Epstein, author of *Healing Visualizations: Creating Health Through Imagery,* found that his patients, even those with physical illnesses, responded best when he prescribed imagery rather than medicine. This approach clearly goes far beyond the usual definitions of psychiatric practice, and the results Epstein describes in his book likewise transcend usual expectations.

Epstein gave a patient with warts an imagery exercise in which the man was to remove his face, turn it inside out, wash it in a crystal-clear, fresh-flowing mountain stream, hang it out to dry in the sun, and then turn it right side out and put it back on, with no warts remaining. This visualization was to be done four times a day for three minutes each time, for a period of three weeks. At the end of that time, the patient's warts were gone.

People with glaucoma, mononucleosis, enlargement of the prostate gland, and numerous other physical ailments experienced similarly impressive healings under Dr. Epstein's guidance. A woman with a fractured bone in her wrist, one notorious for healing slowly, used an Epstein imagery exercise called "Weaving the Marrow," in which she visualized the broken bone and then pictured "white marrow carried in blue channels of lights flowing through the red bloodstream, seeing the arterioles flowing back and forth between the two ends, forming a woven net that brings the two ends closer." She then visualized the two ends knitting together perfectly. Her orthopedist was stunned to discover that the bone had healed fully after three weeks. The usual healing time is three months.[5]

Directed and Nondirected Methods

How can you use this encouraging information in your own healing process? There are many books available on affirmations and visualization. *You Can Heal Your Life* by Louise Hay and *Creative Visualization* by Shakti Gawain are among the best known. Likewise, the books I've mentioned by Drs. Simonton and Epstein offer excellent visualization methods. (See Appendix for sample visualization exercises.)

But before beginning your own visualization work, there are some important questions to consider. First and foremost is this: Is it always appropriate and necessary to visualize a particular, detailed outcome? Most of the literature on the use of affirmations and visualization, including the Simonton and Epstein work we've just seen, assumes that specificity of imagery is all-important. But this may not be the only way to harness the powers of the mind for healing.

Medical philosopher Larry Dossey, M.D., suggests that there are two main ways of doing affirmations and visualization—directed and nondirected. The directed approach is the one utilized by Simonton, Epstein, and most other recent writers on the subject.

With the directed method, you aim for maximum feasible specificity. If you are visualizing an end to your lower back pain, for example, you would learn as much as possible about the anatomy and physiology of the area, and then visualize in great detail the restoration of smooth gliding motion between the vertebrae and the easy and relaxed stretching and contraction of the muscles. You might also picture the blood vessels in the area swiftly transporting toxins away for efficient elimination through the urinary system.

As Simonton's work demonstrates, this directed approach can be very effective. But it is not the only way. You could also choose, as an alternative, to enter a deeply relaxed, meditative state and then surrender to the will of God with an affirmation such as "Thy will be done." (A nonreligious alternative could involve entering the relaxed state and then affirming your oneness with all life and asking Mother Nature to enfold you in her arms.) As part of a non-directed approach, you might also ask to be restored to health in order to have the opportunity to do works of service for others.

Dossey cites a set of highly unusual double-blind experiments in which directed and nondirected methods were used in an attempt to influence simple living systems. The researchers measured parameters like the growth rate of sprouts, after groups of directed and nondirected "prayer practitioners" attempted to influence these processes, each with their respective methods. The directed group was able to increase the growth rate, but the nondirected group was more than twice as effective.[6] Dossey theorizes that directed strategies are most appropriate for extroverted, assertive people, while nondirected strategies are best for introverted, self-reflective individuals. He urges each person to find his or her own way and not to feel compelled by "authorities" to follow any set of rules.

"Most of the books being written in this culture on how to visualize, image, and pray are being written by extroverts," Dossey said when I interviewed him. "If you're someone who is introverted by nature, and you don't feel that comfortable telling God how to fix a problem, you've got a lot of scientific data on your side. There are people who, when they're sick, would just as soon commit to the Absolute, and go up like a jungle cat, crawl into a cave, and wait to see what happens. On the other hand, if you are someone who really needs to be aggressive, specific, and energetic, you've got data on your side, too. Both approaches are successful."[7]

In determining which approach to pursue, there is an additional factor I think is worth considering. It may well be that not all people think alike. The developers of Neurolinguistic Programming hold that most people are primarily visual in their thought patterns, while others are mainly auditory, and still others orient their awareness most easily through the kinesthetic sense (touch). This theory makes a great deal of sense to me, since I am someone who is less visually oriented than most.

For those who do function primarily in a visual mode, specific, directed visualization is made to order. But a substantial number of people, perhaps because they are in the auditory or kinesthetic minorities, find it more difficult to visualize specifically. For them, attempts to perform detailed visualizations can prove a source of great frustration.

Worst of all, if they are unaware that the nondirected method exists and assume that specific visualization is the only choice available, they may decide to opt out of the process altogether at potentially great cost to their health. Just as left-handed people should not be forced to become right-handed for the convenience of others, I feel that auditory, kinesthetic, and introverted people should be informed of alternatives to assertive, sight-oriented visualization methods.

Edgar Cayce on Visualization

The Edgar Cayce readings address the directed vs. nondirected question numerous times. Cayce recommended the use of specific visualization for one reason only—physical healing for oneself. He also frequently recommended healing prayer for others, seeing it as an act of value and service, but he emphasized that healing prayer for others should be done only in a nondirected fashion.

Cayce's stance is consistent with the work of Simonton and Epstein. It is not in agreement, however, with methods in many of the popular books on visualization and affirmations, in which readers are advised to use these methods not only for healing themselves, but for visualizing everything from buying a fancy car to finding a spouse. The Cayce readings consider this to be a form of idolatry.[8]

This is a highly charged, controversial topic in some circles, and this book is not the place to air out the debate in detail. I just wish to make it clear that while I recommend visualization exercises for self-healing purposes, I am not endorsing adaptations of the technique for less high-minded purposes.

Healing from a Distance:
A Scientific Study on Healing Prayer

It will come as a surprise to many that a randomized, double-blind study, published in a mainstream medical journal,[9] demonstrated that prayer had a profound, statistically significant healing effect on hospitalized heart patients. I first learned about this study at a talk by Larry Dossey. Here is Dossey's description from his book, *Meaning and Medicine*:

"Dr. Randolph Byrd, a cardiologist and faculty member of the University of California Medical School at San Francisco, studied almost 400 patients who were admitted to the coronary care unit of San Francisco General Hospital. Most of the patients had had or were suspected of having had a heart attack. They were divided roughly into two groups. Both received state-of-the-art medical care; however, one group was prayed for as well. Their first names and brief sketches of their condition were given to various Protestant and Catholic prayer groups throughout the United States, who were asked to pray for them.

"This was a double-blind study, meaning that neither the nurses, physicians, nor patients knew who was and who was not being prayed for. This meant that preferential care could not unconsciously be given by the health care professionals to one group; nor could the prayed-for group 'try harder' to get well, knowing that they were being prayed for. Neither was one group sicker than the other; there were no statistical differences in the severity of illness between the two groups.

"When this meticulous study was over, the prayed-for group appeared to have been given some 'miracle drug.' They did better clinically in several ways:

"(1) They were far less likely to develop congestive heart

failure, a condition in which the lungs fill with fluid as a consequence of the failure of the heart to pump properly (eight compared to twenty patients).

"(2) They were five times less likely to require antibiotics (three compared to sixteen patients), and three times less likely to need diuretics (five compared to fifteen patients).

"(3) None of the prayed-for group required endotracheal intubation, in which an artificial 'breathing tube' is inserted in the throat and attached to a mechanical ventilator, while twelve of the other group required mechanical ventilatory support.

"(4) Fewer of the prayed-for group developed pneumonia (three compared to thirteen).

"(5) Fewer of those prayed for experienced cardiopulmonary arrest requiring resuscitation (CPR; three compared to fourteen).

"(6) None of the prayed-for group died, compared to three deaths among those not prayed for (this difference was not statistically significant)."

After describing Byrd's amazing study, Dossey comments:

"If the therapy being evaluated had been a new drug or surgical procedure, it would undoubtedly have been heralded as a medical breakthrough. Even a noted skeptic of 'psychic healing,' Dr. William Nolen, author of *The Making of a Surgeon*, remarked [after reading this study] that perhaps physicians should be writing in their orders, 'Pray for my patient three times a day.'"[10]

When I asked Dossey what conclusions he thought were justified by Byrd's study, he said:

"At a bare minimum, the study is very strongly suggestive that prayer has a phenomenal effect, that it has a life-and-death influence on people, even when they do not know they are being prayed for. This is good old classic Caycean action at a distance."[11]

Conscious efforts to use the power of the mind as an aid to healing are an important part of the emerging holistic paradigm, perhaps the most important part. The true miracles of healing occur because a profound shift has occurred within the individual, not only on a physical level, but much deeper. The most important aspects of healing have to do not only with the disappearance of physical symptoms, but with the transformation of mind and spirit. I believe that the degree to which a society recognizes this is an excellent marker for determining the state of its cultural evolution and advancement.

EPILOGUE

TOWARD A
SUSTAINABLE FUTURE

It is no secret that our health care system is in crisis. Costs have spiraled upward, driven by increasing dependence on expensive, high-tech medical and pharmaceutical interventions. I believe that the natural healing practices discussed in this book are an important part of the solution to our current problems. Not overnight, but gradually, over perhaps two or three generations.

If natural diet, regular exercise, meditation/relaxation methods, and other self-healing processes are learned as a normal part of growing up and reinforced by health practitioners and if destructive practices like smoking and substance abuse can truly be curtailed, then the need for high-tech, end-game medicine may eventually diminish to the point where it is small enough to be part of a sustainable system.

The natural healing arts, with chiropractic prominent among them, are by their very nature sustainable. Chiropractic is essentially a low-tech method that can function comfortably in either high-tech or low-tech settings. Its fundamental tools are the hands, heart, and mind of the doctor. While modern chiropractors do avail themselves of high-tech diagnostic (and in some cases therapeutic) methods, these are secondary, not the essence of the art. The essence is the hands-on chiropractic adjustment, which is perfectly sustainable. It is a pure person-to-person interchange, requiring few if any tools.

Being sustainable is not in and of itself a sufficient goal, however. A healing art must also show itself to be effective. It must demonstrate that it has sufficient value to be worth sustaining. I believe this book has made a strong case that chiropractic is both effective and sustainable.

Considering the current state of our health care system, it is quite challenging to envision a grand-scale shift to a sustainable, holistic paradigm. Yet what other sustainable model is being proposed in its place?

Low-cost, low-tech self-care and professional-care methods must play a central role in any health care system that will be sustainable over the long term. This shift in emphasis from present-day disease control to a wellness model promises to significantly improve the overall health of our population.

Unless we make these changes, our society may soon conclude that economic pressures require seriously limiting access to particular high-cost medical procedures and pharmaceutical drugs, even ones that are life-saving for certain people. Or these may be limited by default to the rich or well-insured, as is frequently the case today.

In the long run, this sort of rationing is a formula for social division and moral collapse. It is urgent that we find another way out of this quagmire.

What's clear to me is that we must direct our central focus toward the natural measures which can bring us the health we all sincerely desire. Machines sometimes save lives, but they are not the wellspring from which the waters of life and health are drawn. Health is best sought through commitment to simple, life-sustaining daily activities.

The strength of our common commitment is the best predictor of our eventual success.

APPENDIX

GUIDED IMAGERY TOOLS

This is the mental imagery process utilized by Dr. Carl Simonton and Stephanie Matthews-Simonton for cancer patients, adapted for general use. One way of using this method is to make a slow-paced tape recording of the directions, to guide you through the process.

(1) Go to a quiet room with soft lighting. Shut the door, sit in a comfortable chair, feet flat on the floor, eyes closed.

(2) Become aware of your breathing.

(3) Take in a few deep breaths, and as you let out each breath, mentally say the word, "Relax."

(4) Concentrate on your face and feel any tension in the muscles of your face and around your eyes. Make a mental picture of this tension—it might be like a rope tied in a knot or a clenched fist—and then mentally picture it relaxing and becoming comfortable, like a limp rubber band.

(5) Experience the muscles of your face and eyes becoming relaxed. As they relax, feel a wave of relaxation spreading through your body.

(6) Tense the muscles of your face and around your eyes, squeezing tightly, then relax them and feel the relaxation spreading through your body.

(7) Move slowly down your body—jaw, neck, shoulders, back, upper and lower arms, hands, chest, abdomen, thighs, calves, ankles, feet—until every part of your body is more relaxed. For each part of the body, mentally picture the tension, then picture the tension melting away, allowing relaxation.

(8) Now picture yourself in pleasant, natural surroundings—wherever feels comfortable for you. Mentally fill in the details of color, sound, texture.

(9) Continue to picture yourself in this very relaxed state in this natural place for two to three minutes.

(10) Create a mental picture of any ailment or pain that you have now, visualizing it in a form that makes sense to you.

(11) Picture any treatment you are receiving and see it either eliminating the source of the ailment or pain or strengthening your body's ability to heal itself.

(12) Picture your body's natural defenses and natural processes eliminating the source of the ailment or pain.

(13) Imagine yourself healthy and free of the ailment or pain.

(14) See yourself proceeding successfully toward meeting your goals in life.

(15) Give yourself a mental pat on the back for participating in your own recovery. See yourself doing this relaxation/mental imagery exercise three times a day, staying awake and alert as you do it.

(16) Let the muscles in your eyelids lighten up, become ready to open your eyes, and become aware of the room.

(17) Now let your eyes open and you are ready to resume your usual activities.[1]

Here are two sample imagery exercises for muscle spasm, from Dr. Gerald Epstein's book, *Healing Visualizations*. He suggests doing them as needed every fifteen to thirty minutes, for two to three minutes each session.

Transparent Fingers

Close your eyes. Breathe out three times and begin, in your imagery, to massage your muscle with your transparent fingers. As you do so, sense the blood flowing through the muscle and see the muscle filling with light from above. While massaging, see the muscle elongating as you tease apart the strands and release the knots. Know that when the light has filled the muscle, the blood is flowing through it freely, the muscle is long and unknotted, and the spasm has gone. Then open your eyes.

The Ice Exercise

Close your eyes. Breathe out three times and see your muscle encased in a block of ice. See the ice melting, knowing that as it melts, the muscle is relaxing. After the ice has completely melted, open your eyes, knowing that the spasm has gone.[2]

NOTES

Chapter 2
Twenty Years of Headaches

1. Boline, P.D. "Chiropractic Treatment and Pharmaceutical Treatment for Muscular Contraction Headaches: A Randomized Comparative Clinical Trial." *Proceedings from the 1991 International Conference on Spinal Manipulation.* FCER. Arlington, Virginia.

2. *Chiropractic in New Zealand,* the report of the New Zealand government's commission of inquiry on chiropractic, was published in 1979.

Chapter 3
Dolores' Full Circle: A Body-Mind Journey

1. Gilbert, J.R. "Clinical Trial of Common Treatments for Low Back Pain in Family Practice." *British Medical Journal,* 1985, Vol. 291, pp. 791-794.

2. Barnett, B. Lewis. *Between the Lines (Reflections of a Family Physician),* pp. iv-v of Preface.

Chapter 5
Angela and the Road Not Taken

1. Moody, Raymond. *Life After Life.* New York: Bantam, 1988.

2. Redwood, Daniel. "Raymond Moody: The Pathways Interview." *Pathways.* December 1990, p. 9.

3. Kokjohn, Schmid, Triano, and Brennan. "The Effect of Spinal Manipulation on Pain and Prostaglandin Levels in Women

with Primary Dysmenorrhea." *Journal of Manipulative and Physiological Therapeutics.* 1992. 15: 279-285.

4. Thomason, P.R.; Fisher, B.L.; Carpenter, P.A.; Fike, G.L. "Effectiveness of Spinal Manipulative Therapy in Treatment of Primary Dysmenorrhea: A Pilot Study." *Journal of Manipulative and Physiological Therapeutics.* 1979. 2: 140-145.

5. Werbach, Melvyn. *Nutritional Influences on Illness,* pp. 184, 364-369.

Chapter 6
David's Bridge

1. Weil, Andrew, M.D. *Natural Health, Natural Medicine,* p. 135.

2. *Ibid.,* pp. 135-136.

3. Puryear, Herbert, and Thurston, Mark. *Meditation and the Mind of Man,* pp. 30-37.

4. Drawn from a variety of Western interpreters of Indian tradition, including Randolph Stone, D.C., D.O., N.D., and Ram Dass (Richard Alpert, Ph.D.).

Chapter 8
Chiropractic: An Alternative Healing Art Enters the Mainstream

1. From internal AMA documents introduced into evidence by the chiropractic plaintiffs at the *Wilk v. AMA* trial. Data from the federally mandated study was to be used to determine whether chiropractic should be included in Medicare, the government-sponsored health insurance program for older Americans. Passage of the Corman-Stone bill in 1973 brought chiropractic services into the Medicare system.

2. Eddy, David M. Quoted in *Chiropractic: A Review of Current Research.* Foundation for Chiropractic Education and Research. Arlington, Va., p.1. Dr. Eddy, a medical physician, is professor of Health Policy and Management at Duke University.

3. Eisenberg, David, et al. "Unconventional Medicine in the United States: Prevalence, Costs, and Patterns of Use." *New England Journal of Medicine.* January 28, 1993. 328: 246-252.

4. Leach, Robert. *The Chiropractic Theories: A Synopsis of Scientific Research,* p. 24. Leach cites as his source an article by Elizabeth Lomax called "Manipulative Therapy: A Historical Perspective from Ancient Times to the Modern Era," which appeared in *The Research Status of Spinal Manipulative Therapy,* published by the United States Government Printing Office (1975), pp. 11-17. This monograph contains the proceedings of a conference on spinal manipulation, convened by the National Institute for Neurological and Communicable Diseases and Stroke (NINCDS).

5. Copland-Griffiths, Michael. *Dynamic Chiropractic Today,* pp. 119-120.

6. *Ibid.,* pp. 121-122.

7. Leach. *op. cit.,* p. 25.

8. Gibbons, Russell. "The Evolution of Chiropractic: Medical and Social Protest in America," in *Modern Developments in the Principles and Practice of Chiropractic,* edited by Scott Haldeman, p. 23.

9. Sharpless, Seth. "Susceptibility of Spinal Roots to Compression Block." In Goldstein, Murray (editor): *The Research Status of Spinal Manipulative Therapy.* Washington, D.C., Government Printing Office, 1975, pp. 155-161.

10. Kirkaldy-Willis, W., and Cassidy, J. "Spinal Manipulation in the Treatment of Low-Back Pain." *Canadian Family Physician.* 1985. 31:535-540.

11. Meade, T.W., Dyer, S., et al. "Low Back Pain of Mechanical Origin: Randomised Comparison of Chiropractic and Hospital Outpatient Treatment," *British Medical Journal,* June 2, 1990. Vol. 300, pp. 1431-1437.

12. Dr. T.W. Meade, interviewed on a Canadian Broadcasting Corporation (CBC) program, as quoted in *Chiropractic: A Review of Current Research.* Foundation for Chiropractic Education and Research. 1992.

13. Koes, B.W.; Bouter, L.M.; et al. "Randomised Clinical Trial of Manipulative Therapy and Physiotherapy for Persistent Back and Neck Complaints: Results of One Year Follow-Up." *British Medical Journal.* March 7, 1992, Volume 304, pp. 601-605.

14. Ebrall, P.S. "Mechanical Low Back Pain: A Comparison of Medical and Chiropractic Managment Within the Victorian WorkCare Scheme." *Chiropractic Journal of Australia.* June 1992, Volume 22, Number 2, pp. 47-53.

15. Jarvis, K.B.; Phillips, R.B.; et al. "Cost per Case Comparison of Back Injury Claims of Chiropractic versus Medical Management for Conditions with Identical Diagnostic Codes." *Journal of Occupational Medicine.* August 1991, Volume 33, Number 8, pp. 847-852.

16. Wolk, S. *Chiropractic versus Medical Care: A Cost Analysis of Disability and Treatment for Back-Related Workers' Compensation Cases.* Foundation for Chiropractic Education and Research, September 1987.

17. Boline, P.D. "Chiropractic Treatment and Pharmaceutical Treatment for Muscular Contraction Headaches: A Randomized Comparative Clinical Trial." *Proceedings from the 1991 International Conference on Spinal Manipulation.* FCER. Arlington, Virginia.

18. North American Spine Society's Ad Hoc Committee on Diagnostic and Therapeutic Procedures. *Spine.* 1991. Vol. 16, No. 10.

19. Davis, H., AV MED Medical Director. Miami, Florida. 1982. The chiropractor was Mark Silverman, D.C. This evidence was presented as part of the *Wilk v. AMA* trial.

20. Cherkin, D., and MacCornack, F. "Patient Evaluations of Low Back Pain Care from Family Physicians and Chiropractors," *Western Journal of Medicine,* March 1989, Volume 150, pp. 351-355.

21. Gilbert, J.R. "Clinical Trial of Common Treatments for Low Back Pain in Family Practice." *British Medical Journal,* 1985, Vol. 291, pp. 791-794.

22. Curtis P., and Bove, G. "Family Physicians, Chiropractors, and Back Pain." *Journal of Family Practice,* November 1992, Vol. 35, pp. 551-555.

23. The Gallup Organization, *Demographic Characteristics of Users of Chiropractic,* 1991.

Chapter 9
Foundations of the Chiropractic Model

1. Copland-Griffiths, *Dynamic Chiropractic Today,* p. 159.
2. Bourdillion, J.F. *Spinal Manipulation,* pp. 205-206.
3. Copland-Griffiths, *op. cit.,* p. 162.
4. Mazzarelli, Joseph, D.C. (editor). *Chiropractic: Interprofessional Research,* pp. 69-76.
5. Yates, R.G.; Lamping, D.L.; Abram, N.L.; and Wright, C. "Effects of Chiropractic Treatment on Blood Pressure and Anxiety: A Randomized, Controlled Trial." *Journal of Manipulative and Physiological Therapeutics,* 1988. 11: 484-488.
6. Kokjohn, K.; Schmid, D.M.; Triano, J.J.; Brennan, P.C. "The Effect of Spinal Manpulation on Pain and Prostaglandin Levels in Women with Primary Dysmenorrhea." *Journal of Manipulative and Physiological Therapeutics,* 1992. 15: 279-285.
7. Thomason, P.R.; Fisher, B.L.; Carpenter, P.A.; Fike, G.L. "Effectiveness of Spinal Manipulative Therapy in Treatment of Primary Dysmenorrhea: A Pilot Study." *Journal of Manipulative and Physiological Therapeutics.* 1979. 2: 140-145.
8. Brennan, P.C.; Kokjohn, K.; Katlinger, C.J.; Lohr, G.E.; Glendening, C.; Hondras, M.A.; McGregor, M.; Triano, J.J. "Enhanced Phagocytic Cell Respiratory Burst Induced by Spinal Manipulation: Potential Role of Substance P." *Journal of Manipulative and Physiological Therapeutics,* 1991. 14: 399-408.
9. Klougart, N.; Nillson, N.; Jacobsen, J. "Infantile Colic Treated by Chiropractors: A Prospective Study of 316 Cases." *Journal of Manipulative and Physiological Therapeutics,* 1989. 12: 281-288.
10. Falk, J.W. "Bowel and Bladder Dysfunction Secondary to Lumbar Dysfunctional Syndrome." *Chiropractic Technique,* 1990. 2: 45-48.
11. Borregard, P.E. "Neurogenic Bladder and Spina Bifida Occulta: A Case Report." *Journal of Manipulative and Physiological Therapeutics,* 1987. 10: 122-123.
12. Masarsky, C.S., and Weber, M. "Screening Spirometry in the Chiropractic Examination." *ACA Journal of Chiropractic,* February 1989. 23: 67-68.

13. Masarsky, C.S., and Weber, M. "Chiropractic and Lung Volumes—A Retrospective Study." *ACA Journal of Chiropractic*, September 1986. 20: 65-68.

14. Hewitt, E.G. "Chiropractic Treatment of a Seven-Month-Old with Chronic Constipation: A Case Report." *Proceedings of the National Conference on Chiropractic and Pediatrics* (International Chiropractors Association), 1992, pp. 16-23.

15. Bachman, T.R., and Lantz, C.A. "Management of Pediatric Asthma and Enuresis with Probable Traumatic Etiology." *Proceedings of the National Conference on Chiropractic and Pediatrics* (International Chiropractors Association), 1991, pp. 14-22.

16. Browning, J.E. " Mechanically Induced Pelvic Pain and Organic Dysfunction in a Patient Without Low Back Pain." *Journal of Manipulative and Physiological Therapeutics*, 1990. 13:406-411.

17. Goodman, R. "Cessation of Seizure Disorder: Correction of the Atlas Subluxation Complex." *Proceedings of the National Conference on Chiropractic and Pediatrics* (International Chiropractors Association), 1991, pp. 46-56.

Chapter 10
Edgar Cayce's Holistic Theories on Manual Medicine

1. Peterson, Barbara (editor). *The Collected Papers of Irwin M. Korr*, pp. 170-175.

2. Edgar Cayce reading 1158-24.

3. Peterson, *op. cit.*, p. 174.

4. *Ibid.*

5. Korr, Irwin. "The Spinal Cord as Organizer of Disease Processes: The Peripheral Autonomic Nervous System." *Journal of the American Osteopathic Association*, October 1979. 79:82-90.

Chapter 11
Diet and Nutrition

1. American Dietetic Association's 1988 position paper on vegetarian diets, quoted in *Dr. Dean Ornish's Program for Reversing Heart Disease*, pp. 261-262.

2. Redwood, Daniel. "John Robbins: Interview." *Coastal Pathways.* June 1991, p. 5.

3. For a detailed examination of Dr. Campbell's study, see *Diet, Life Style, and Mortality in China: A Study of the Characteristics of Sixty-Five Chinese Counties*, published by Cornell University Press in 1990.

4. Reilly and Brod, *The Edgar Cayce Handbook for Health Through Drugless Therapy*, p. 67.

5. Edgar Cayce reading 5148-1.
6. Edgar Cayce reading 1158-31.
7. Edgar Cayce reading 3180-3.
8. Edgar Cayce reading 3386-2.
9. Edgar Cayce reading 3118-1.
10. Edgar Cayce reading 3542-1.
11. Edgar Cayce reading 4047-1.
12. Edgar Cayce reading 137-30.
13. Edgar Cayce reading 900-393.

Chapter 12
Exercise and Yoga

1. Paffenbarger, et al. "Work Activity of Longshoremen as Related to Death from Coronary Heart Disease and Stroke." *New England Journal of Medicine*, 1970. 282:1109-14.

2. Paffenbarger, R., et al. "A Natural History of Athleticism and Cardiovascular Health." *Journal of the American Medical Association*, 1984. 252:491.

3. Paffenbarger, R., et al. "Physical Activity, All-Cause Mortality, and Longevity of College Alumni." *New England Journal of Medicine*, 1986. 314:607-9.

4. Murphy, *The Future of the Body*, pp. 425-431.

5. Blair, Kohl, Paffenbarger, et al. "Physical Fitness and All-Cause Mortality." *Journal of the American Medical Association.* 1989. 262:2395-2401.

6. Ornish, Dean. *Dr. Dean Ornish's Program for Reversing Heart Disease*, p. 324.

7. Edgar Cayce reading 1968-9.
8. Edgar Cayce reading 2090-2.

9. Edgar Cayce reading 578-5.

10. Redwood, Daniel. "Swami Satchidananda." *Venture Inward.* July 1989, p. 32.

11. Edgar Cayce reading1523-2.

12. Edgar Cayce reading 4462-1.

13. Edgar Cayce reading 470-37.

14. Satchidananda, Sri Swami. *Integral Yoga Hatha,* pp. 11-25.

15. Edgar Cayce reading 4520-4.

16. Edgar Cayce reading 288-38.

17. Reilly, Harold. *The Edgar Cayce Handbook for Health Through Drugless Therapy,* p. 113.

18. Edgar Cayce reading 2072-5.

19. Edgar Cayce reading 2533-3.

Chapter 13
Meditation and Relaxation

1. Dienstfrey, Harris. *Where the Mind Meets the Body,* p. 31.

2. Murphy and Donovan, *The Physical and Psychological Effects of Meditation,* p. 27.

3. *Ibid.,* p. 30.

4. *Ibid.,* pp. 15-18.

5. Brown, D.P., and Engler, J. "The Stages of Mindfulness Meditation: A Validation Study." *Journal of Transpersonal Psychology,* 1980, 12 (2), 143-192.

6. McEvoy, T.M.; Frumkin, L.R.; Harkins, S.W. "Effects of Meditation on Brainstem Auditory Evoked Potentials." *International Journal of Neuroscience.* 1980. 10:165-170.

7. Pagano, R.R., and Frumkin, L.R. "The Effect of Transcendental Meditation on Right Hemisphere Functioning." *Biofeedback and Self-Regulation,* 1977, 2 (4), 407-415.

8. *Ibid.*

9. Benson. *The Relaxation Response,* pp. 162-163.

10. Easwaran, Eknath. *Meditation,* p. 71.

11. Chopra, Deepak. *Unconditional Life,* p. 161.

12. Redwood, Daniel. "The Pathways Interview: Deepak Chopra." *Pathways.* December 1991, pp. 5-7.

13. *Ibid.,* p.7.

14. Chopra, *op. cit.*, p. 190.
15. Edgar Cayce reading 281-41.
16. Puryear, *Healing Through Meditation and Prayer*, pp. 4-5.
17. *Ibid.*, p. 6.
18. Edgar Cayce reading 1861-19.

Chapter 14
Visualization, Affirmations, and Prayer

1. Simonton, O. Carl, et al. *Getting Well Again*, p. 77.
2. *Ibid.*, p. 11.
3. Simonton and Hansen. *The Healing Journey*, p. 5.
4. Spiegel, D.; Kraemer, H.C.; Bloom, J.R.; and Gottheil, E. "The Effect of Psychosocial Treatment on Survival of Patients with Metastatic Breast Cancer." *Lancet*. October 14, 1989. Vol. II (8668): 888-891.
5. Epstein, Gerald. *Healing Visualizations*, pp. 12-13.
6. Dossey, Larry. *Recovering the Soul*, p. 58.
7. Redwood, Daniel. "The Pathways Interview: Larry Dossey." *Pathways*. March 1992, p. 29.
8. Edgar Cayce reading 705-2.
9. Byrd, Randolph. "Positive Therapeutic Effects of Intercessory Prayer in a Coronary Care Unit Population," *Southern Medical Journal*. 1988. 81:7, pp. 826-829.
10. Dossey, Larry. *Meaning and Medicine*, pp. 182-183.
11. Redwood, *op. cit.*, p. 27.

Appendix
Guided Imagery Tools

1. Simonton, Simonton, and Creighton. *Getting Well Again*, pp. 131-136.
2. Epstein, Gerald. *Healing Visualizations*, p.151.

BIBLIOGRAPHY

Chiropractic and Manual Medicine

Bourdillion, J.F., M.D. *Spinal Manipulation.* 3rd ed. New York: Appleton Century Crofts, 1982.

Copland-Griffiths, Michael, D.C. *Dynamic Chiropractic Today: The Complete and Authoritative Guide to This Major Therapy.* Wellingborough, U.K.: Thorsons, 1991.

Cort, Andrew, D.C. *Your Healing Birthright: Taking Responsibility for Ourselves and Our Planet.* Rochester, Vt.: Healing Arts Press, 1990.

Ford, Clyde, D.C. *Where Healing Waters Meet: Touching Mind and Emotion Through the Body.* Barrytown, N.Y.: Station Hill Press, 1989.

Haldeman, Scott, D.C., M.D., Ph.D., editor. 2nd ed. *Modern Developments in the Principles and Practice of Chiropractic.* New York: Appleton Century Crofts, 1992.

Leach, Robert, D.C. *The Chiropractic Theories: A Synopsis of Scientific Research.* Baltimore: Williams and Wilkins, 1986.

Palmer, Daniel David. *The Science, Art, and Philosophy of Chiropractic.* Davenport, Iowa: Palmer College of Chiropractic, 1910.

Strang, Virgil, D.C. *Essential Principles of Chiropractic.* Davenport, Iowa: Palmer College, 1984.

Holistic Medicine and the Mind-Body Connection

Chopra, Deepak, M.D. *Ageless Body, Timeless Mind.* New York: Harmony Books, 1993.

Chopra, Deepak, M.D. *Perfect Health: The Complete Mind-Body Guide.* New York: Harmony Books, 1990.

Chopra, Deepak, M.D. *Quantum Healing: Exploring the Frontiers of Mind/Body Medicine.* New York: Bantam, 1989.

Chopra, Deepak, M.D. *Unconditional Life: Discovering the Power to Fulfill Your Dreams.* New York: Bantam, 1991.

Dientsfrey, Harris, Ph.D. *Where the Mind Meets the Body.* New York: Harper Collins, 1991.

Dossey, Larry, M.D. *Meaning and Medicine: Lessons from a Doctor's Tales of Breakthrough and Healing.* New York: Bantam, 1991.

Dossey, Larry, M.D. *Recovering the Soul: A Scientific and Spiritual Search.* New York: Bantam, 1989.

Epstein, Gerald, M.D. *Healing Visualizations: Creating Health Through Imagery.* New York: Bantam, 1989.

Gordon, James, M.D. *Holistic Medicine.* New York: Chelsea House, 1988.

Gordon, James, M.D., and Rosenthal, Raymond, M.D. *The Healing Partnership.* Washington: Aurora, 1984.

Kabat-Zinn, John, Ph.D. *Full Catastrophe Living: Using the Wisdom of Your Body and Mind to Face Stress, Pain, and Illness.* New York: Delacorte, 1991.

Moyers, Bill. *Healing and the Mind.* New York: Doubleday, 1993.

Shealy, C. Norman, M.D., Ph.D. *90 Days to Self-Health.* Columbus, Ohio: Ariel Press, 1976, 1987.

Shealy, Norman, M.D., and Myss, Carolyn. *The Creation of Health.* Walpole, N.H.: Stillpoint Publishing, 1988.

Siegel, Bernie, M.D. *Love, Medicine, and Miracles.* New York: Harper and Row, 1986.

Weil, Andrew, M.D. *Health and Healing.* Boston: Houghton Mifflin, 1983, 1988.

McGarey, William, M.D. *Healing Miracles: Using Your Body Energies.* San Francisco: Harper and Row, 1988.

Mein, Eric, M.D. *Keys to Health: The Promise and Challenge of Holism.* San Francisco: Harper and Row, 1989.

Pagano, John, D.C. *Healing Psoriasis: The Natural Alternative.* Englewood Cliffs, N.J.: The Pagano Organization, 1991.

Reilly, Harold, D.Ph.T., D.S., and Brod, Ruth. *The Edgar Cayce Handbook for Health Through Drugless Therapy.* New York: Macmillan, 1975.

Stearn, Jess. *The Sleeping Prophet.* New York: Bantam, 1967.

Sugrue, Thomas. *There Is a River.* Virginia Beach: A.R.E. Press, 1942, 1992.

Diet and Nutrition

Ballentine, Rudolph, M.D. *Diet and Nutrition.* Honesdale, Pa.: Himalayan Publishers, 1978.

Diamond, Harvey and Marilyn. *Fit for Life.* New York: Warner Books, 1985.

Gerber, James, D.C. *Handbook of Preventive and Therapeutic Nutrition.* Gaithersburg, Md.: Aspen Publishers, 1993.

Haas, Elson, M.D. *Staying Healthy with Nutrition.* Berkeley, Calif.: Celestial Arts, 1992.

Haas, Elson, M.D. *Staying Healthy with the Seasons.* Berkeley, Calif.: Celestial Arts, 1981.

Kushi, Michio. *The Book of Macrobiotics: The Universal Way of Health and Happiness.* Tokyo: Japan Publications, 1977.

Lappe, Frances Moore. *Diet for a Small Planet.* Rev. ed. New York: Ballentine Books, 1987.

Lappe, Frances Moore, and Collins, Joseph. *Food First: Beyond the Myth of Scarcity.* New York: Ballantine, 1977, 1979.

Murray, Michael, N.D., and Pizzorno, Joseph, N.D. *Encyclopedia of Natural Medicine*. Rocklin, Calif.: Prima Publishing, 1991.

Null, Gary. *The Vegetarian Handbook: Eating Right for Total Health*. New York: St. Martin's, 1987.

Ornish, Dean, M.D. *Dr. Dean Ornish's Program for Reversing Heart Disease*. New York: Random House, 1990.

Ornish, Dean, M.D. *Eat More, Weigh Less*. New York: Harper Collins, 1993.

Pfeiffer, Carl, Ph.D. *Mental and Elemental Nutrients: A Physician's Guide to Nutrition and Health Care*. New Canaan, Conn.: Keats Publishing, 1976.

Robbins, John. *Diet for a New America*. Walpole, N.H.: Stillpoint Publishing, 1987.

Serrentino, Jo. *How Natural Remedies Work*. Point Roberts, Wash.: Hartley and Marks, 1991.

Satchidananda, Sri Swami. *The Healthy Vegetarian*. Buckingham, Va.: Integral Yoga Publications, 1986.

Shurtleff, William, and Aoyagi, Akiko. *The Book of Tofu*. New York: Ballantine, 1979.

Weil, Andrew, M.D. *Natural Health, Natural Medicine*. Boston, Mass.: Houghton Mifflin, 1990.

Werbach, Melvyn, M.D. *Nutritional Influences on Illness: A Sourcebook for Clinical Research*. New Canaan, Conn.: Keats Publishing, 1987.

Wright, Jonathan, M.D. *Dr. Wright's Book of Nutritional Therapy*. Emmaus, Pa.: Rodale Press, 1979.

Cookbooks

Brown, Edward Espe. *Tassajara Bread Book*. Rev. and updated ed. Boston: Shambhala Publications, 1970, 1986.

Colbin, Annemarie. *The Book of Whole Meals*. New York: Ballantine, 1979, 1983.

Diamond, Marilyn. *The American Vegetarian Cookbook from the Fit for Life Kitchen.* New York: Warner Books, 1990.

Gelles, Carol. *Wholesome Harvest.* New York: Little, Brown and Co., 1992.

Madison, Deborah, with Edward Espe Brown. *The Greens Cook Book.* New York: Bantam, 1987.

Robertson, Laurel; Flinders, Carol; and Godfrey, Bronwen. *The New Laurel's Kitchen: A Handbook for Vegetarian Cooking and Nutrition.* Berkeley, Calif.: Ten Speed Press, 1976, 1986.

Sahni, Julie. *Classic Indian Vegetarian and Grain Cooking.* New York: William Morrow, 1985.

Shulman, Martha Rose. *Fast Vegetarian Feasts.* Rev. ed with Fish. New York: Doubleday, 1982.

Shulman, Martha Rose. *Mediterranean Light: Delicious Recipes from the World's Healthiest Cuisine.* New York: Bantam, 1989.

Shulman, Martha Rose. *The Vegetarian Feast.* New York: Harper and Row, 1979.

Somerville, Annie. *Fields of Greens.* New York: Bantam, 1993.

Walters, Lynn. *Cooking at the Natural Foods Cafe in Santa Fe.* Freedom, Calif.: The Crossing Press, 1992.

Yoga and Exercise

Brena, Steven, M.D. *Yoga and Medicine: The Reunion of Mind-Body Health and the Meaning of Yoga Concepts with Modern Medical Knowledge.* New York: Julian Press, 1972.

Murphy, Michael. *The Future of the Body: Explorations into the Further Evolution of Human Nature.* Los Angeles: Jeremy P. Tarcher, 1992.

Satchidananda, Sri Swami. *Integral Yoga Hatha.* New York: Holt, Rinehart and Winston, 1970.

Meditation

Benson, Herbert, M.D. *The Relaxation Response.* New York: William Morrow, 1975.

Murphy, Michael, and Donovan, Steven. *The Physical and Psychological Effects of Meditation: A Review of Contemporary Meditation Research with a Comprehensive Bibliography* 1931-1988. San Rafael, Calif.: Esalen Institute, 1988.

Murphy, Michael. *The Future of the Body: Explorations into the Further Evolution of Human Nature.* Los Angeles: Jeremy P. Tarcher, 1992.

Puryear, Herbert, Ph.D., and Thurston, Mark, Ph.D. *Meditation and the Mind of Man.* Rev. ed. Virginia Beach, Va.: A.R.E. Press, 1988.

Puryear, Meredith Ann. *Healing Through Meditation and Prayer.* Virginia Beach, Va.: A.R.E. Press, 1978.

Herbs and Herbal Medicine

Kowalcik, Claire, and Hylton, William. *Rodale's Illustrated Encyclopedia of Herbs.* Emmaus, Pa.: Rodale Press, 1987.

Murray, Michael, N.D. *The Healing Power of Herbs: The Enlightened Person's Guide to the Wonders of Medicinal Plants.* Rocklin, Calif.: Prima Publishing, 1992.

Murray, Michael, N.D., and Pizzorno, Joseph, N.D. *Encyclopedia of Natural Medicine.* Rocklin, Calif.: Prima Publishing, 1991.

Messegué, Maurice. *Of People and Plants.* Rochester, Vt.: Healing Arts Press, 1973, 1991.

Serrentino, Jo. *How Natural Remedies Work.* Point Roberts, Wash.: Hartley and Marks, 1991.

Tierra, Michael, L.Ac. *The Way of Herbs.* New York: Pocket Books, 1983.

Teeguarden, Ron. *Chinese Tonic Herbs.* New York: Japan Publications, 1987.

Weil, Andrew, M.D. *Natural Health, Natural Medicine.* Boston, Mass.: Houghton Mifflin Company, 1990.

Energy Medicine

Becker, Robert, M.D., and Selden, Gary. *The Body Electric: Electromagnetism and the Foundation of Life*. New York: William Morrow, 1985.

Becker, Robert, M.D. *Cross Currents: The Perils of Electropollution, the Promise of Electromedicine*. Los Angeles: Jeremy P. Tarcher, 1990.

Connelly, Dianne, Ph.D., M.Ac. *Traditional Acupuncture: The Law of the Five Elements*. Columbia, Md.: The Centre for Traditional Acupuncture, 1979.

McGarey, William, M.D. *Healing Miracles: Using Your Body Energies*. San Francisco: Harper and Row, 1988.

Siegel, Alan, N.D. *Polarity Therapy: The Power That Heals*. San Leandro, Calif.: Prism Press, 1987.

Smith, Fritz Frederick, M.D. *Inner Bridges: A Guide to Energy Movement and Body Structure*. Atlanta: Humanics Limited, 1986.

Inspirational Personal Stories of Healing

Asistent, Niro Markoff. *Why I Survive AIDS*. New York: Fireside/ Simon and Schuster, 1991.

Breslow, Rachelle. *Who Said So?* Berkeley, Calif.: Celestial Arts, 1991.

Schneider, Meir. *Self-Healing: My Life and Vision*. New York: Routledge and Kegan Paul, 1987.

INDEX

A

American Dietetic Association 150
American Holistic Medical Association (AHMA) 132
American Journal of Physiology 190
American Medical Association 103
amitriptyline 24
amnesia 73
anecdotal evidence 104
antibiotics 3
antihistamines 22, 60
arthritis 7, 31, 167
aspirin 30
asthma 2, 3, 60, 126, 145
  and low blood sugar 60
auditory mode of perception 208
Ayurveda 132, 138

B

Barnett, B. Lewis 46
beans 153
bed rest 40
beer 99
"bellows breathing" 188
Benson, Herbert 190, 195
Bhagavad-Gita 200
Bible 200
bicycle riding 55, 168
bioflavonoids 160
Blair, Steven 167
blood pressure
  and diet 34
  decrease from exercise 164
  high 31, 191
    and diet 153
  improvement in 33
blood sugar
  abnormalities 33
  levels 27
blood supply
    44, 85, 91, 124, 171, 172, 177

Body, Mind, and Sugar 60
bonesetters 106
Bourdillion, J.F. 124
Bove, Geoffrey 117
brain scans 38
brain-wave coordination 192
breathing
  alternate nostril 186
  as cleansing process 186
  conscious 186
  effects of exercise 164
  exercises 90, 186, 188
  forceful 187
  improvement in 33
  slow and deep 187
  voluntary or involuntary 186
British Medical Journal 113, 115
bronchitis 7
Buffalo, State University of New York 5
Byrd, Randolph 209

C

caffeine 27, 147, 154
calcium, deposits in ligaments 122
Campbell, T. Colin 151
camphor 63
Canadian Family Physician 112
cancer
  and diet 156
  and visualization 203
  and Western diet 150
  breast 150, 153
    and protein intake 151
    effects of counseling 205
  colon 150, 153
    and protein intake 151
  effects of exercise on incidence 164
  lung 145, 150

musculoskeletal system 122
music 5, 6, 8
mutuality 46, 47

N

National Cancer Institute
146, 151
national health insurance
13, 34
natural healing 5, 6, 7, 8
natural healing arts 213
natural healing philosophy
10, 74, 105
*Natural Health, Natural
Medicine* 89
nausea 64, 72, 97
near-death experience (NDE)
69
nervous system 23, 44, 121
and respiration 90, 91
autonomic 124
cerebrospinal 137
energy centers 95
parasympathetic 91, 140
and atlas vertebra 91
and yoga 173
supply to lungs 91
supply to stomach 98
vagus nerve 91, 123, 137
phrenic nerve 91
sympathetic
23, 137, 138, 190
and blood vessels 90
and brain-wave patterns
141
and conditioned reflexes
141
as amplifier 140
as junction of mind and
body 141
as overall tuning mecha-
nism 140
elevated blood pressure
190

head-and-neck exercise
172
increased heart rate 190
increased oxygen
consumption 190
increased respiratory rate
190
need for broad view of
141
nerves supplying ear 124
origins 23
osteopathic research
139, 142
overrides muscle fatigue
140
pathways to head 123
relation to cerebrospinal
system 140, 141
supply to lungs 90
supply to stomach 98
wide-ranging role 140
Neurocalometer (NCM) 138
Neurolinguistic Programming
207-208
New Zealand report 34
niacin 154
nicotine 85, 90, 92
and the brain 90
as stimulant 90
effects on blood vessels 85
North American Spine Society
116
Novalis 12
numbness
31, 38, 75, 79, 123
arm 76
feet 75
hand 75
leg 39, 72
pelvic 48, 53, 54
pinwheel testing 31
nuts and seeds 27, 61, 154

O

obesity 150
Of People and Plants 8
Office of Alternative Medicine
    197
"one cause-one cure" 108
"one white crow" 169
orange peels 160
Ornish, Dean
    146, 149, 165, 167
    reversal diet 153
orthodoxy, danger of 95, 96
osteoarthritis 135
osteopathy
    49, 52, 76, 107, 133, 136,
    138, 141, 142, 173
    beginnings 107
    early twentieth century 133
osteoporosis 150
    and diet 153
    and protein intake 151
outcomes research 104, 105
outside intervention, limits of
    9
oxygen deprivation 70

P

Paffenbarger, Ralph 164
pain 123
    abdominal 36, 43, 56, 74
    ankle 128
    as possible contraindication
        for exercise 173
    causing embarrassment 22
    chronic 49, 50
    ears 70
    elbow 128
    foot 75
    groin 56
    hip 72, 74, 128
    knee 128
    leg 38

    lower back
        7, 35, 61, 75, 76,
        79, 85, 90, 92
    menstrual 73, 79
    neck 20, 54, 84
    related to urination 56, 59
    shoulder 72, 74, 84, 128
    upper back 84
    visualization for 206
    wrist 128
Palmer, B.J. 110
Palmer College of Chiropractic
    8, 9, 10, 13, 122, 138
Palmer, Daniel David xviii,
    8, 107, 108, 109, 124, 135
pancreas 157
paradox 83
    knowledge and wisdom 96
Paré, Ambroise 106
paresthesia 75
    definition 31
Pathways 15, 16
patient satisfaction
    research data 116
peanuts 27, 29
pecans 99
physical therapy 9, 73
    machines 9
pleurisy 3
pneumonia 3
polarity therapy
    11, 41, 43, 77, 78, 94, 138
    neck contact, 86
    right-left balance 87, 88
    sensation of heat 86
    specific contacts 77, 78, 88
positive thinking 45, 203
posture 57
poultry 65
practicing medicine without a
    license 109
prayer 207
    groups 209
    scientific study 209
premenstrual syndrome 93

Advance Praise for *A Time to Heal*

Dr. Redwood has provided a superb summary of the emerging consensus favoring the inclusion of chiropractic and other holistic concepts as part of a comprehensive approach to healing. This is now almost universally recognized by thinking health professionals, and it is essential if we are going to reverse the stagnation created by excessive modern technology.

As Dr. Redwood has amply acknowledged, manipulative therapy goes back almost 5,000 years. I consider it one of the great tragedies of the medical profession that the latter rejected manipulative therapy when it was introduced in America a century ago. Now is the time to fully recognize its value.

—C. Norman Shealy, M.D., Ph.D., founding president, American Holistic Medical Association; author, *90 Days to Self-Health* and *The Creation of Health*

Dr. Daniel Redwood has pulled together information from many sources, including the Edgar Cayce readings, in such a way that this book becomes an easily read and yet thought-provoking manuscript. He has incorporated the material into his life and profession in such a way that he speaks from a depth of knowledge and experience which makes the reader understand the practicality of the material and also its inspirational value.

I believe this is the best interpretation and understanding of the Edgar Cayce material in relation to chiropractic that I have seen, and I highly recommend it to anyone who is interested in learning more about the chiropractic profession, the Edgar Cayce material, and how these can be used in our lives.

—Gladys McGarey, M.D., former president, American Holistic Medical Association; author, *Born to Live*

Dr. Redwood has clearly demonstrated his thorough understanding of the term "holistic healing" in this comprehensive volume. More important, he knows how to convey it most effectively to his readers. This work is a "must" for anyone interested in expanding his or her knowledge of the subject.

—John O.A. Pagano, D.C., author, *Healing Psoriasis: The Natural Alternative*

At a time when the issue of health care is before the Congress and the American people, this book could not be more timely. A Time to Heal is engagingly easy to read. I came away with an ex-

panded appreciation for the value and scope of chiropractic as an alternative health care modality.

I especially enjoyed the specific suggestions offered by Dr. Redwood that encourage and empower the reader to take greater responsibility for his/her own health by incorporating periods of deep relaxation into daily life.

—Steven Halpern, Ph.D., recording artist and
composer; author, *Sound Health*

In this day of accelerating medical change, Daniel Redwood's A Time to Heal *will add to the momentum.*

A fine essay on the possible which in conventional medicine is considered impossible.

—J.N. Wu, L.Ac., chairman, District of Columbia
Acupuncture Advisory Board; translator, *Ling Shu*
(*The Yellow Emperor's Inner Classic*) and *Yi Jing*
(*Book of Changes*)

By discussing chiropractic in the context of the larger holistic health movement, Dr. Redwood takes the reader far beyond the "sprain and strain" concept of the field. The chapter, "Chiropractic: An Alternative Healing Art Enters the Mainstream" is a fascinating, uncluttered read, while still managing impeccable scientific and historical accuracy. Dr. Redwood's discussion of the diagnostic logic which guides doctors of chiropractic in their clinical work is excellent. In general, this is the finest book on chiropractic for the lay reader that we have ever read.

—Charles Masarsky, D.C., and Marion Weber, D.C.,
co-editors, *Neurological Fitness*

With unique clarity and intimacy, Daniel Redwood has written a wonderfully readable book. He has been able to bring forth in a new light the health teachings of Edgar Cayce and then integrate them with emerging concepts on body-mind-spirit healing and wholeness. I would recommend this book for everyone.

—Sandra McLanahan, M.D., director of stress
management training, Preventive Medicine
Research Institute

What Is A.R.E.?

The Association for Research and Enlightenment, Inc. (A.R.E.®), is the international headquarters for the work of Edgar Cayce (1877-1945), who is considered the best-documented psychic of the twentieth century. Founded in 1931, the A.R.E. consists of a community of people from all walks of life and spiritual traditions, who have found meaningful and life-transformative insights from the readings of Edgar Cayce.

Although A.R.E. headquarters is located in Virginia Beach, Virginia—where visitors are always welcome—the A.R.E. community is a global network of individuals who offer conferences, educational activities, and fellowship around the world. People of every age are invited to participate in programs that focus on such topics as holistic health, dreams, reincarnation, ESP, the power of the mind, meditation, and personal spirituality.

In addition to study groups and various activities, the A.R.E. offers membership benefits and services, a bimonthly magazine, a newsletter, extracts from the Cayce readings, conferences, international tours, a massage school curriculum, an impressive volunteer network, a retreat-type camp for children and adults, and A.R.E. contacts around the world. A.R.E. also maintains an affiliation with Atlantic University, which offers a master's degree program in Transpersonal Studies.

For additional information about A.R.E. activities hosted near you, please contact:

A.R.E.
67th St. and Atlantic Ave.
P.O. Box 595
Virginia Beach, VA 23451-0595
(804) 428-3588

A.R.E. Press

A.R.E. Press is a publisher and distributor of books, audio-tapes, and videos that offer guidance for a more fulfilling life. Our products are based on, or are compatible with, the concepts in the psychic readings of Edgar Cayce.

We especially seek to create products which carry forward the inspirational story of individuals who have made practical application of the Cayce legacy.

For a free catalog, please write to A.R.E. Press at the address below or call toll free 1-800-723-1112. For any other information, please call 804-428-3588.

A.R.E. Press
Sixty-Eighth & Atlantic Avenue
P.O. Box 656
Virginia Beach, VA 23451-0656